THE END OF THE TWINS

Saul Diskin

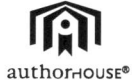

authorHOUSE®

AuthorHouse™
1663 Liberty Drive
Bloomington, IN 47403
www.authorhouse.com
Phone: 1-800-839-8640

Published by AuthorHouse 2/29/2012

ISBN: 978-1-4685-3014-8 (sc)
ISBN: 978-1-4685-3015-5 (e)
ISBN: 978-1-4685-3013-1 (hc)

Library of Congress Control Number: 2011962642

CONTENTS

BROOKLYN AND BEYOND

To be an identical twin is to be outside the realm of normal, ordinary human experience. It is to be more than one person and to be incomplete at the same time. It is both to live in the public gaze, especially when very young and indistinguishable from the other twin and at the same time to have an existence intensely private, foreign and unknowable to everyone else, including parents. It is to be helpless before the stares and gawks of adults, but at the same time, from the earliest age, to know, and sometimes relish, the power to draw their attention. It is to suffer the unsolicited and usually unwelcome ministrations of the curious but also the ability to unnerve them when they see two human beings who are identical. It is, in short, to be a superior freak.

A child cannot know these things. But even as little children my twin brother Martin and I knew that we were looked upon as different. Adults, trying to comprehend the phenomenon, were initially unnerved when they saw us. Hiding a certain disorientation, they were almost always friendly, even delighted. "Look at them. How cute. How sweet." Because we were two discrete human beings who looked exactly alike, a somewhat rare phenomenon, an understanding seemed to exist that permitted even strangers to take liberties. The adult eye darted from one twin to the other searching for distinguishing characteristics. That behavior has changed very little from the time of our youth. Even as adults strangers would not hesitate to address us in the third person, seeing us not as persons, but as a phenomenon. Looking directly at us, unabashedly, not even pretending to soften the intrusion, the same polite adult whose eyes would avert at the sight of an amputated limb or other physical deformity, would say in a loud voice, "Look at that. You can hardly tell them apart. It's incredible.

Hold your head a little that way. I think I can tell them apart. That one doesn't have a scar on his cheek, do you? Let's see. Can your wives tell you apart?"

As children, on our teeming Brooklyn street, our mother, called us home, bawling out the window, "Marty Sauly, Sauly Marty." From the distance even she couldn't tell us apart.

We were closer than can be easily described, too close. We knew what the other was thinking, experiencing. Not in the popular way of understanding. We could not read each others thoughts specifically, but we knew how the other was feeling, precisely. We knew the meaning of every gesture, of every body attitude, of every facial expression, of every grimace. We could tell when a joke was coming and the laughter would start before the words were out. Our play was synchronous. We could enter effortlessly in the other's imaginary world. Marty and I breathed the same air and although we didn't make a deliberate effort to monitor the other's activities and whereabouts, we always knew what the other was doing and where he was. Waking from a nap one would look through the bars of his crib and see his brother a few feet away, eyes open, staring at his brother. No acknowledgment was necessary: each of us was simply seeing a permanent and unchanging part of his environment. We were two cubs in the same genetically determined cage. Our environment, at least in our early years, was virtually identical. For a time it was the two of us against the world, sharing praise in our successes, comforting each other in our failures and defending each other against outside intrusion. We were one person walking around in two little bodies.

Breathing heavily, sweating and anxious, I rest on the third floor landing of the five-story Brooklyn walkup. My burst of nervous energy spent itself racing up the stairs. I am following Marty to the roof, a dangerous and forbidden place where neither had ever ventured. Our mother, unaware of where we were, sits on a folding chair in a sliver of shade on the crowded sidewalk below, talking with other women. She would be furious if she found out. Alone and frightened, I resignedly place my sweating forehead against the cool tiled wall. It is summer and I am dressed as all five-year olds: high topped shoes, scuffed and torn beyond repair, short pants, and a polo shirt. My black hair, shorn to the scalp in June to discourage head lice, had grown thick enough to begin curling. The dim yellow glare from the bulb overhead shines malevolently through the broken fixture. The air, redolent with cabbage, chickenfat, garlic and onions, the odors of eastern European Jewish kitchens, hangs still and heavy on the landing. Muffled cries of youngsters at play filter up from the street, completing my feeling of isolation. In the summer all life is out in the street, only fear and danger lurk within the dark and humid interior.

"Where's Marty? Why did he go to the roof without me? What will he do up there? He didn't even tell me he was going. Why didn't he wait for me? How did he get there?" To give myself courage I concentrate on the pattern of little gray octagonal tiles set within the border of the smooth white granite, the same material as the stair risers. It is no use. With one hand on the worn banister, I resume trudging up the stairs. I have to find Marty. I begin to cry. I don't know exactly how to get to the roof. I have never been this high on the stairs before. I am not even sure who lives on the upper floors.

The last flight ends at the heavy metal door to the roof. There is no landing, no overhead light. The only light is the sickly remnant from the lower landing. The door has no knob. "How do you open it?" Whimpering, in desperation, I push against it. It opens slowly. The bright midday light surges in and the expanse of tarry roof opens to my sight. There is Marty! He is near the edge, smiling and waving at me. I smile, tentatively, relieved at finding him, my tears drying. My mood turns quickly, the evidence of my eyes telling me that Marty is safe, that we are together. The newly discovered terrain of the roof is appealing, exotic. It is full of adventurous possibilities for us. Together we can do anything. Abruptly, Marty lifts himself jerkily up to the top of the parapet, his body lunging forward. "What are you doing? Marty, Marty!"

Beyond Marty there is nothing but sky. He is slowly elevating, a tiny profile against the limitless, brilliant background. He is rising, so slowly. The huge drifting clouds form bizarre, changing shapes, imaginary animals and landscapes in silver and gray. They are beckoning Marty, drawing him gently off his feet, off the roof, away from me. He is happy. He looks at me briefly, his face wide with wonder and joy, and leaning over the parapet, calls, "Mommy, Mommy" toward the sidewalk five stories below.

I stand, fixed, the warm tar a sluggish river carrying me at its pace, preventing me from flying to Marty and grabbing him tightly to hold him on the parapet. I know I will watch helplessly while Marty falls from the roof and sucks me along in his wake. A current of acid is inside my stomach, hurting me, poisoning me. Marty's legs leave the floor of the roof, dangling unconcernedly, merrily. My stomach is in convulsion. My mind, numb to everything else in the world except my brother, sees clearly that in the next instant his legs will get higher and higher and with the parapet as fulcrum, make a short, slow, graceful topple over the edge. Forced to watch, I will see him falling, his face twisting into a grimace of fear as he realizes in midair that it is too late,

3

that there is no remedy, no undoing. He will think, "Where's Sauly, where's Mommy, where's Daddy?" Then he will hit the ground, making the sound that Mommy makes, crushing the head of a fish in her teeth. Where's Marty? No more Marty. No more twins.

When our mother reached the roof, wild with worry and ready to thrash us both, she found me dazed and silent. I had thrown up. They told me my stomach had "turned." For days after the roof incident I couldn't keep food down. Marty and I were skinny little things and the fear was that I would sicken or die from malnutrition and anemia. I was put into a hospital for a couple of weeks where they fed me through tubes. I could barely walk when they allowed me to come home. For days after Mom wheeled me around in a baby stroller. When we had meat, the bloody juice was reserved for me, to "build up my blood."

When I recall that episode now, more than half a century later, I don't have to try to remember what I thought about my twin brother dying… my churning stomach tells me.

It is a common characteristic of eastern European Jews, whether from *shtetl* or city, that family history extends only as far back as the memory of the oldest living family member. Marty and I, and later Phil, our younger brother, knew about our family's history from those stories. When we were young they were offered as flashbacks, told to us as nostalgic recollections, without point, not as instruction. Later, when we were older and our family's past was of interest to us, we asked questions, sometimes receiving answers. Some of that past, particularly of our father's family, was too painful for him to discuss voluntarily.

Dad's people came from just outside Kovno, in Lithuania. His father had been a truck farmer. Because he was a Jew he was not permitted to own land. He survived by leasing small parcels, about half of them sandy soil and the other half clay. In a dry year the clay land produced well and the crops on the sandy land burned up. In a wet year the crops on the sandy land did well and the crops on the clay land rotted. Dad's father died before the First World War. During the war, Dad, his three siblings who had not emigrated to America and his mother were banished from their home by an edict of the Czar. The Czar feared, probably correctly, that the Jews of the region, having suffered unspeakably, would collaborate with the Germans, who were advancing toward the East. In 24 hours they were required to leave the region. Dad recalled bitterly having to load sacks of potatoes on the wagon that carried him and his mother to exile. His siblings were loaded on trains to meet them later. The trains never stopped and Dad never saw them again. Years later he found out from relief organizations that his sister had been transported to Siberia. His brother with his wife and three children were shipped to the Ukraine where they all starved to death. He never determined the fate of his youngest brother.

Marty and I were born in Harlem in the middle of the Depression. Our parents lived in a building they always referred to as the cooperative, a place hospitable to immigrants with leftist leanings. There, in Yiddish and Russian and Polish and rudimentary English and finally believing they were out of the reach of the Czar, safe from the Cossacks and pogroms, they dreamed of the downfall of the capitalist system and of organizing a more just society. They talked of global events with greater urgency and fervor than of the daily life around them. Gradually, though, their revolutionary zeal was dulled by what they considered betrayal by their idols, coupled with a general increase in their personal fortunes. The Depression finally gave way to better times and the erstwhile bombthrowers became small businessmen, shopkeepers, jobholders with better prospects, even householders. The beginning of our father's disillusionment came with the Stalin show trials of the Mensheviks. The Hitler Stalin Pact completed his conversion.

We moved from Harlem to the Bronx. The Depression still lingered like a chronic disease. Our father was working but still not making ends meet. The same was true of our mother's sister, Aunt Leda and Uncle Jack. To economize on rent the two families shared a house in a semi-rural part of Brooklyn. Marty and I were too young to remember the house, but as mother told us about it years later she shuddered. The place was overrun with rats and one day she found one nosing about our sleeping bodies. Later, we both became deathly ill, having been poisoned, it was thought, by some substance in the house. Shortly thereafter, in the late thirties, Dad found steady work as a knitter on Jacquard machines in the sweater trade and we were able to move to Union Street.

Union Street must have resembled a brighter, more modern Moldavanka, the Jewish ghetto in Odessa where my mother came from. There were people everywhere. The apartments were small and everyone, it seemed, had children and elderly, immigrant parents, unable to fend for themselves in the new world. Like a squeezed balloon full of water, indoor life flooded out into the street. In the summertime the women unfolded chairs on the sidewalk so they could watch their children as they visited with neighbors, interrupting the conversation occasionally to help those children on the cusp of being toilet trained. The girls were held up over the street with their legs spread, the mother standing daintily on the sidewalk, bent slightly toward the street, eyes scanning to ward off salacious glances. The boys were engulfed by their mothers, fumbling for their penises, all the while making sounds that folklore suggested aided the urination process.

Peddlers would lead their horses through the street, parting the throng of punchball and stickball players. They were working their routes, these horse-drawn fruit and vegetable stores. The more enterprising specialized in summer delicacies, perhaps an entire wagon load of watermelon or cantaloupe. Mother would open a melon in the apartment, never in the street, and always make the same pronouncement,"Not bad, but not an *Odessa dinyeh.*" (a melon from Odessa). She was glad to be in this country. She had suffered enough in Odessa, but her memory magnified the delight of the fruits grown in Bessarabia. The new country could never produce a peach as sweet as the one from home. It was the last grudging pining for the home she was torn from.

The children lived in the street in the summer and in the winter until the cough everyone seemed to develop grew too intense and the cold too bitter. Ranging from kindergarten age, like Marty and me, to early teens, there were games for all. The street was reserved for the gutter games, using the manhole covers as home plate and second base, and if cars were parked on the street their fenders were used for first and third base. The sidewalks were the courts for skelly, tickets, jump rope, hopscotch and stoopball. And throughout this hive, *ringaleevio* was played, a form of hide-and-seek in which the pursued could hide anywhere: behind seated women, lampposts, cars, in the basements, and when chased, between people or gameplayers. The mothers' nightmare was that a darting child would be struck by a car and it happened from time to time. We heard that a boy who had hitched his sled to a bus on Utica Avenue was killed. He had not reckoned on the airbrakes when the transition was made from trolley cars to busses and he slid under the rear wheels and was crushed. We didn't actually know the boy. He lived on the next block.

The block we lived on, between Utica Avenue and Schenectady Avenue, a residential street, was a canyon of elevatorless apartment houses. No trees, no flowers, just brick buildings and concrete sidewalks and asphalt street.

The most important commercial street, Utica Avenue, was still paved in cobblestones. Tiny shops lined the street, purveying goods to satisfy most human needs. At the din-filled, chaotic bazaar on Utica, within a block or two of Union Street, one could buy food, clothing, furnishings, sporting goods, tobacco, newspapers and drugs. Most offerings shared one common characteristic. Everything, except food, was cheap. Goods had to be to be affordable to the working people of Union Street. Food was a different story. There was no compromise for just the right chicken for the Friday night meal or the right combination of smoked fish and cheeses for the Sunday morning breakfast, one of the few meals of the week in which the father of the house joined his family. A piece of lamb could not be too old for a stew; a beet for borscht could not have lain around too long, a peach not too soft, a carrot not discolored. In the quest for the perfect ingredient the dialogue between the shopkeepers and the housewives would reach loud and angry heights. The price of the food was one thing, the quality another.

For Marty and me Union Street was a pleasurable pandemonium. There was constant movement, people thronging everywhere. As the adults passed they had a smile for us. We were secure, protected, unafraid.

Early on a summer evening, Marty and I were playing on the fringe of the big boys' punchball game. The ball eluded one of the fielders and rolled to Marty. A boy, very tall for his perhaps sixteen years, ran toward him and commanded him to throw the ball to him so that he might have the chance, illegally, to throw the runner out at home. Gleefully, but unintentionally, Marty threw the ball over his head. Enraged, the boy advanced on Marty and slapped him to the ground at the precise moment that Dad, coming from the subway, rounded the corner from Utica Avenue. Dad went from a composed stroll to a dead run with no intermediate steps. The big boy fled, his long arms and legs flailing for survival, as the short, dark, barrel-chested immigrant, his newspaper still under his arm, chugged after him, eating up the distance between them, a cold look of murder in his eye. The boy escaped to the basement and the back yard beyond and over the fence to the next street. Dad had to give up the chase, but he knew who the boy was as we all did. Marty and I were frightened that the boy would hurt us when Dad wasn't around to protect us. We were also somewhat terrified at how angry Dad became. It was obvious to us, even as children, that he had lost control and we feared for what he might do.

The boy was summoned to court to answer my father's complaint. He stood on one side of the bench, flanked by his parents. On the other side of the bench stood our family. Dad glared at the boy. He seemed to be coiled, ready to attack and dismember the young criminal no matter the penalty he would face. Marty and I prayed it would be over soon and prayed equally fervently that Dad would not stutter so badly he would not be understood.

The judge looked down from the bench, his face drawn into dark wrinkles, his bushy eyebrows curling to attention. "Where are the two boys involved? Stand there, in front of me." Dad took Marty by the shoulder pushing him toward the center of the bench. The boy that slapped Marty was a hundred pounds heavier and eighteen inches taller.

"You honor, my son is only fiftin years old."

"Are you his lawyer?"

"I'm de faddah. I got a summons to bring him in court."

"Well, I'm the judge. I say who talks and who doesn't and when. You understand?"

"Yeah."

"What?"

"Yes, you honor."

"What's your name, son?"

Marty wrapped his arm around Dad's thigh and Dad held him close by the shoulder. "Martin Diskin," he said, quietly.

"These are your parents? Who is that over there? Is that your brother? What's his name? Hey, wait a minute. He looks just like you. Are you twins?" The judge swung his head from Marty to me and back, an avuncular smile lighting his face.

"Yes. His name is Saul Diskin."

"And you, the defendant, your name is Franklin Abramowitz?"

"Yes, your honor," he said, his head down, in a tremulous voice.

"Look at me when you speak and speak loud enough so I can hear you."

Franklin raised his head and repeated his answer. He was trembling and the red pimples on his cheeks were glistening.

"As I understand from the report, Franklin, you slapped Martin hard enough to knock him down to the sidewalk. You didn't give him any warning. There was no provocation, you just ran over to him and slapped him. Is that right?"

"We were playing punchball and the batter punched the ball over my head and Marty got it and threw it over my head so I couldn't even throw the runner out."

"Wait a minute. Before I ask you again whether you hit Martin, tell me this. If he hadn't been there the ball would have rolled much further and you would have had no chance to get it in time to throw the runner out. Is that right?"

"You honor, dis is abot punchball?"

"Mr. Abramowitz, where are you from?"

"Poland."

"Did you play much punchball in Poland?"

Mr. Abramowitz, his hard, large hands clumsy in repose, looked toward the ceiling and breathed deeply, audibly. "No, you honor."

"Then have the goodness not to interrupt me anymore while I am questioning your son. I'll give you time to talk when I'm finished." Mr. Abramovitz lowered his head and glared sideways at his son. His eyes said, *'When I get you home I'll teach you to cost me a day's pay.'*

"Now, Franklin, just tell me, yes or no, did you slap Martin down to the sidewalk?"

Franklin's "Yes", was more an exhalation than a word, a weary, frightened sibilance.

"So, first you were prepared to cheat at punchball, to keep the ball in play that was stopped by someone not in the game. I was a two-and-a-half sewer hitter when I was a kid in Brownsville, and I still know the rules. You know as well as I do that if someone on the sidewalk stops a fairly hit ball the runner takes an extra base. But you got so mad that Martin didn't cooperate with your cheating you hit him hard enough to injure him. You are very lucky that Martin was not seriously hurt. But this shows what kind of a boy you are. Your first instinct is to hit someone half your size."

Franklin's shoulders started shaking. Tears came to his eyes.

"Look at me, Franklin. I could send you away to reform school where you would be with boys your own size who might want to do to you what you did to Martin just for the sport of it. Do you want me to do that?"

"No, *Schloime*, don't let him do dot," screamed Mrs. Abramovitz. Franklin was sobbing, clutching his father.

"Mrs. Abramowitz, calm yourself. I'm not going to do it this time. I am going to return him to your home and I want you to keep an eye on him, keep him out of trouble. If he comes back to court again, off to reform school with him. Now, Franklin, I want you to look at Martin and shake his hand and tell him you're sorry and that you won't do it again. Martin, I want you to shake Franklin's hand, okay? And Mr. Abramowitz and Mr. Diskin, shake each others hand and we'll put an end to all of this."

Franklin's white sweating hand engulfed Marty's small, dark hand. He was contrite and relieved and grateful for the outcome. The men touched each others hand as if each contained something putrefied. Their eyes did not meet. Each, in turn, offered their stretched hand over the top of the bench to the judge, who shook them both. Both families left in separate directions.

Marty and I were exultant. Franklin would not bother us. The judge guaranteed that. And Dad did all of this without exploding, without hitting anyone and without his face contorting with stutters. Despite it being a working day we stopped at a luncheonette and Dad ordered an egg cream. Marty and I knew that it meant that he would give us each a sip. We waited in excited anticipation, too short to see the drink's preparation. We could hear the sound the tall glass made as it was plopped onto the marble counter top, though muffled by the overflow of the milk and seltzer and chocolate syrup, it was the sound of priceless luxury, the sound of foretold pleasure. We could hear the satisfied sigh Dad made after he sipped the drink and with a mirth-surpressed secret glance between us we knew it would be a second or two before he would lower the glass to one of us saying, "Drink it slowly, it's cold."

We moved. Not to another city or neighborhood, but further down Union street, near Schenectady Avenue. It felt like a different city to Marty and me. It was less noisy, less crowded, the gateway to a calmer atmosphere, to tree-sentried streets, single family houses, propertied people, car owners. The best was that it was around the corner from a public library, available to us without having to cross a street. As soon as we could we marched to the library with Mom to sign up for our own cards. From then on we could go to the library without her. We attended readings at the library given by women who dressed well and who spoke in soft tones with no trace of a foreign accent. These were real Americans.

Marty and I were in the second grade. Proficient readers by then, we dispatched our school assignment in minutes, and then the real reading began. We coursed through Grimm's fairy tales with hungry excitement, graduating to Norse myths and then to a children's edition of Beowulf. We devoured other folk tales, adventure stories, tales of pirates, stories of high imagination. The rule was that one had to keep books for at least a week. Driven to finish the books we had checked out before the end of the week, we invariably completed reading them a day or two earlier. That day or two was agony for us and when the week's end came around we raced to the library holding the books to be returned, our spirits wild with joy at the prospect of yet more books to read the following week.

One evening Dad came crashing through the door to the apartment lugging a cardboard carton tied with a heavy rope. He put it down on the living room floor, a smile glowing on his face. We surrounded the box as Dad painstakingly began to untie the knot which had tightened on its journey up the stairs. The rope would not be cut. It was of one piece and would be saved.

"What's in the box? Is it for us?'

"You'll see, just wait till I untie it."

Dad licked his thumb, the one with the cracked nail, and with his stubby mawls of fingers, dug into the heart of the knot.

"Is it toys for us?" we asked, crowding Dad. We knew it was a silly question. A toy was bought for us once a year around New Years at a store on Utica Avenue. Dad continued smiling but did not respond. Mom came out of the kitchen and watched in the background. Marty and I twitched around the carton, careful not to bump Dad. By now it was confirmed that whatever treasure lay concealed in the box would soon be ours.

"Mommy, what is it?" we whined impatiently.

"I don't know. Moish, hurry up."

Dad flashed an unsmiling look at her as he made the final assault on the knot. His fingers had found the most secure purchase he could get and he clamped the loop end. His bicep flew to attention. We held our breath as he pitted his fingers against the knot. Either the knot or his finger would break soon. His hand trembled. From the slightly relaxed movement we knew the knot had given way and the loose end was being pulled through the coil. Deliberately, without hurrying, he pulled the remainder of the rope through the slip knot and, accompanied by the ratcheting sound of the rope rubbing roughly against the cardboard, the rope was free and the top of the carton rose slightly.

"Open it and look," Dad said, satisfiedly.

There were books, dozens of them, and they were ours, not the library's. They were very used books, the kind bought by the pound or rescued before someone threw them away. Many of the bindings were broken, pages were marked and missing, but they were ours. The Bobsey Twins, Nancy Drew, The Hardy Boys, a book about dolphins, geography books, Bomba The Jungle Boy, the collected works of Kipling. We were weak with happiness. Now we could finish our library books on Wednesday, even Tuesday, and have reading until the Thursday we went to the library.

Marty and I did virtually everything together. We arose in beds separated by two feet, dressed exactly alike and ate breakfast together, complaining with equal fervor about the mandatory dose of cod liver. We went to the same school, the same classroom. After school we came home together and either played with the same friends in the street or read books together, lying on our bellies on the floor next to each other. We got into mischief together, were punished or spanked together. Whatever one learned the other knew shortly thereafter. When we discussed something new we forged the differences of opinion into one jointly held view, not because one's views prevailed over the others, but because our thinking was so similar. We learned together and taught each other about the world and as our two intelligences, our two curiosities grew and strengthened an ache set in that presaged the break with each other that we would soon have to make.

Despite the intense closeness we had developed, or perhaps because of it, it was there in that second apartment on Union Street, when we were about eight years old, that our rivalry began.

Our younger brother Phil was born while we lived in that apartment. Perhaps that had something to do with it: the realization that twins were not the only form of child. Phil, after all, was our brother, our parents' son, and yet he was not our age or size. Phil's arrival may have made Marty and I understand that no sibling could be as close to either of us as we were to each other. We may also have concluded that, judging from our parents' response to Phil and our observation of our friends, all singletons, that our relationship and status was unusual.

We felt the deficiency of lacking uniqueness. The confusion that others exhibited when they encountered us in turn confused us about our own identity. If adults could not tell the difference between Martin and Saul, then was there indeed any difference? Were we separate human beings or were we creatures that had only a partial existence, needing abilities and strengths of the other to survive? Without the novelty that the world accorded us could we distinguish ourselves? We would have to part to find out.

Everything confirmed that judgment. Rhoda and Moish, our Mom and Dad, now had three children but they only seemed to refer to two entities, Phil and the Twins. Were the two of us only worth one of Phil? These are speculations. Those events are too far in the past to pretend that the memories are either accurate or objective. What is certain is that at around the time that Phil was born Marty and I began having disagreements about many things. The subject of the disagreement was never important. It could involve a book both wanted to read, a punishment one suffered for a transgression of the other, a humiliation one visited on the other. These proximate irritants were fanned by a torture too subtle for outsiders, even our parents, to fully understand the cruelty of. And we were equally skilled at inflicting it on the other.

It involved feigning danger to himself. A common form was when our mother would take us on a subway journey. The malicious one would walk close to the edge of the platform, especially when the sound of the oncoming train would grow louder. The other one would squirm and suffer, begging and insisting that our mother order the other one back from the edge. The torturer would ogle the sufferer, exulting momentarily in the power he exercised. The pain the onlooker experienced had to do with the impotence he felt by not being able to alter the event that could lead to his brother's destruction. The taunter was in complete control. If he lost his footing while aping and teasing at the platform's edge and fell into the path of the oncoming train he would take the other, standing apart, holding Mommy's hand, with him. We could not tell where one ended and the other began. The victim of that episode would store the hurt and settle the score at the next fight.

Martin had a bad eye from an accident at about the age of six. A sliver of glass from a milk bottle we were demolishing with a hammer cut his cornea. He was taken to a neighborhood hospital where, as our family legend went, a visiting German eye surgeon performed an emergency operation on him, saving him from blindness that would have resulted from scarring on the cornea. Although the vision in the affected eye was so bad that the big E on the eye chart remained a blur, he compensated well enough with his good eye so that he served in the army and became an academic, which required him to read a great deal. Later in life I needed reading glasses before he did.

As a child I was a stutterer, like our father. Those deficiencies, Marty's bad eye and my stuttering were almost always the precipitant, the insult drawn from our arsenal, which would assure the onset of hostilities. I would make fun of his bad eye, he would lampoon my stuttering. Soon after the taunting began we would fly at each other with murder in our hearts. We beat each other with fists and knees and elbows. We choked each other, we punched, we sought to do serious injury to the other. Because we were so evenly matched physically, the winner invariably was the one who felt the greatest outrage at the taunts that, by that time, neither one remembered.

Late one winter afternoon when we were perhaps nine years old, Marty and I, for an unremembered cause, began one of our marathon fights. It started in the dark hallway where we had been playing and migrated to the cramped living room in our small apartment. The dirty winter dusk had sucked all the light out of the room. The electric lights were not on yet and Marty and I, under cover of the vanishing light, alternately attacked and retreated until the furniture began to bang around and our mother roared into the room from the kitchen. Never shrinking from physicality, she waded into the middle of our battle shouting threats and dispensing punches and kicks. At last Marty and I parted. Struggling to catch our breath and standing five feet apart with hands knotted into fists, we faced each other with looks of fiery hatred. The moment Mom left the room we flew at each other, strengthened by the short rest. She pulled us apart again and yet again we resumed the battle as soon as she left. At last, unable to pull us apart, she pronounced the worst upon us, an operatic *maledizione*, "I'll tell Daddy when he comes home and you'll get it." We were beyond caring. We continued, although exhaustion was rendering our choke holds less viselike and our punches slower and less painful when they landed. Dad arrived while we were still fighting. Mother came rushing out of the kitchen to tell him what we had been doing for well over an hour and bade him put a forceful end to it. He looked at us, still furiously engaged, and on his way to his dinner, said, "They'll stop when they're tired enough."

Seen from my current, aging vantage, it seems plain that the anger and violence assisted in what we were undergoing. Stronger than reason, a feeling, a tropism, both informed and drove our young minds and bodies to cast off the comfortable protection of twinhood and seek something unknowable and frightening to us...separation. We had to do it. We didn't know why or how. We never discussed it, never. Creating the boiling rivalry between us made the separation easier. The more we competed with each other, the greater the rancor between us grew and the more we could differentiate one from the other. For the first time in our lives we deliberately cultivated different interests. It made the inevitable parting bearable.

We moved from Union Street to Crown Street, four blocks away. Marty and I entered the third grade. Crown Street felt like the country to Marty and me. Our side of the street had five story walkups, one of which we lived in, interspersed with single and two family houses, known by us as "private houses." Our side of the street had small elm trees, protected by iron grates and each apartment house had shrubs planted in front of it. Every one of the private houses had some planting, even a little lawn between the sidewalk and the porch. On the entire other side of the street stood a private hospital whose long driveways flanked a large, hilly lawn bordered by what to us were elaborate ornamental plantings. On the sidewalk along the entire frontage were sycamore trees, large and stately, that in full leaf shaded their entire side of the street and halfway to our side. They were the tallest trees around and everyone felt proud of them. When they were uprooted during a hurricane in the late forties, tearing the concrete sidewalks up with them, there was a palpable sense of loss in the neighborhood.

We lived on Crown Street until we both left home some eight or nine years later. During that time we completed the process of separation. For the first time in our lives we began to form separate friendships. We went to school and back home together but after school we could go back to the school playground, the schoolyard we called it, and there we became interested in and broadened our ability in sports. It was barely two blocks from our house and a place our mother let us go unsupervised whenever we wanted. The schoolyard had a regulation basketball court, a softball diamond, room for touch football or stickball, and hand ball against the bordering apartment house wall.

As little boys and newcomers to the neighborhood we mostly had to watch and retrieve stray balls. We waited to use the courts until the big boys were through and while we waited we imbibed the culture of sports. We heard the worshipful discussions of professional sports: batting averages, points or touchdowns scored, ERA's, yards gained or lost, wins and losses among prizefighters, breeding and performance of racehorses, and which teams in any given sport had the best chances. Arguments quickly turned bitter and violent, some to be resolved only with fists. If the discussions about sports had a hard edge, engaging in the schoolyard form of those sports had an even harder edge. Many of those contests, principally basketball and softball, were played for wagers, the winning team keeping the stakes. At many of those contests, melees broke out. A hard elbow thrown, a pitch hitting a batter, a disputed call always seemed to be the proximate cause. A push, a shove, would sometimes result in a fight involving fists and sometimes bats, between a dozen of the big boys or, as we called them after the war, the "veterans."

Marty and I, two skinny, black haired, browneyed, dark skinned boys at nine and ten and eleven watched this bad temper, this aggression, and accepted it as normal behavior. It was not much different at home. When Mom and Dad had an argument it would escalate quickly. Words were hissed or spat or stuttered at each other, until shortly the New York Times would be smashed down on the table, Dad uttering the crack-of-doom expletive, "Ah fah Chrissake." Fear would seep into every corner of the apartment. No one was safe in approaching him in those moments. He usually stalked out of the house to calm down in the evening air while the rest of us were relieved that a crisis had been averted temporarily. The aftermath of such incidents was usually a black silence in which Dad would not speak to Mom, sometimes for many months.

Mom was quicker to forgive, but more volatile. She didn't seem to have patience for subtleties. If the situation wouldn't yield to an easy answer, she wanted to smash it. She was quick with a smile or a slap or a kiss or a loud angry word. Redheaded, with a white, freckled complexion, she was strong and solid. She didn't hesitate supporting the position she took with physical action. We couldn't discuss anything with her. Her answers were final. She represented her knowledge of the world as absolute and would tolerate no contradiction.

Before we entered first grade Dad taught us the soliloquy from Hamlet. From time to time he hoisted one of us onto the kitchen table to show us off to a neighbor or friend. Raising us swiftly from floor to table in his strong arms he beamed as we rewarded him with our performance. Sometimes at night, when he thought we were asleep, he read epic Russian poems aloud, without stuttering, his voice crackling with drama, his arms sawing the air.

Dad was ruminative, thoughtful, patient with a problem. When we first learned to play chess we eagerly challenged him. We always regretted it. Instead of the hasty moves we made, he pondered as if he were in a grandmasters tournament without the time constraints. I watched his darkly handsome face as he concentrated on the board, his hooded, Asiatic eyes revealing nothing of his thinking. Deliberately, his eyes not leaving the board, he licked his finger ritually and drew deeply on his Chesterfield. He wasn't a particularly good chess player, always seeming to be searching for an answer, a truth that ever eluded him, never completely accepting an obvious solution.

When Mom and Dad were at peace with each other and when things were going well at school and at play and between Marty and me and Phil, the household was full of comfort and a sense of adventure and controlled wildness that pleased us all. But those conditions were rare.

It was in that atmosphere, that Marty and I began the slow and painful process of separation in earnest. We tried to outdo the other in contests of every kind. Not just to surpass the other, not just to hit the ball further in punchball or stickball or score more in basketball or hit better or make better fielding plays in softball, but to humiliate the other, to embarrass the other in front of our contemporaries. Then, at the end of a day of ranks and insults, we would go home to the same house and fight it out with a rage born of hurt that no outsider ever saw and with the sickening fear of the day when we would part.

I became friends with Robert Silverberg. New to our neighborhood, he was put into our fourth grade class in the middle of the year. Almost two years younger than most of the children, he was of a different social and economic class than the rest of us. Both of his parents worked and were professionals, his mother a teacher and his father an accountant. He had a live-in maid, a light skinned black woman from the south named Lottie.

Robert was smarter and, though younger, more worldly than the rest of us, and he let us all know it. As a result he was bullied liberally. I was smaller than most of the other boys and would let no slight pass without strong comment. Robert and I became the target of at least one of the same bullies. Perhaps that was the common ground that brought us together initially. Later, it was our interest in science fiction, which we began to read at about the same time.

For a time Robert and I published a science fiction magazine, *Spaceship*, which we heliographed, assembled and sold to doting relatives. Robert was my friend, not Marty's. Most of the time I would go to his house, only occasionally to mine. Because he was an only child, his apartment was spacious, clean, uncluttered, and, I thought, luxuriantly appointed. His mother, American born, was austere and unsmiling. I believed she found me an unsuitable playmate for Robert.

Perhaps I considered his circumstances exotic: parents who spoke without accents, a more affluent life style, the only servant in the neighborhood. And Robert himself, unabashedly interested in the life of the mind. It was a glimpse of something foreign to the atmosphere of polyglot immigrants who worked with their hands that I was used to. I would not share that relationship with Marty. The rest of the life Marty and I shared centered around school, schoolyard, street and home. He had no exclusive friendships at that time. He would have to wait till he started high school. Together, Robert and I studied Esperanto, attempted to simplify Latin grammar, and write science fiction. We went to the same high school, but there our interests diverged. He continued diligently pursuing intellectual interests and science fiction. He went to college and later to a highly successful career as a science fiction writer. I drifted.

Just after the war, Dad, who was then about 50, bought his first car, a 1939 Nash Ambassador. Gathered in our small kitchen on Crown Street on a spring evening, Mom, Phil, Marty and I surrounded Dad and the seller of the car, the principals in the transaction. Under our serious, watchful eyes Dad squeezed out the limp, soiled bills, 50's and 20's, and let them fall gently to the oil-clothed table in an unruly pile, as leaves from a tree on a windless late autumn day. We were thrilled that Dad was buying a car. It was his car, not the family's car. Even Mom, referring to the machine only in the feminine, called it his car. Detroit, after gearing up for wartime production, had not yet returned to manufacturing for the civilian market and cars were at a premium, probably $1,000 for this one. But that was all right. Dad could afford it. He was, by now, a skilled mechanic on Jacquard machines and worked steadily for good wages.

In an uncharacteristic outburst of optimism that the peacetime prosperity would continue, Mom and Dad agreed on a vacation at Lena's, a rustic resort in Connecticut. This was not a Catskills *kochalein*, a crude bungalow in which you did your own cooking, equipped with an icebox and sometimes only an outhouse. There were, we were told, activities for us: swimming, Ping-Pong, volley-ball, trips to a large boating and fishing lake. And, instead of the trip we all dreaded; crawling in an endless line of hired cars and choking on the overheated gasoline fumes amid the angry parental admonition to hold one's head out the window when one of us puked, we drove in our own car. The children were thrilled to be adventuring over the concrete ribbon that slashed through the clean smelling, undulating and green countryside: a far and exotic destination. Mom treated the entire enterprise as a harbinger of success for our family. She discussed it as if it were a guilty secret.

We had two rooms, one for Mom and Dad, when he came on weekends, and the other for Marty and Phil and me. For the month of our stay, Mom did not have to cook or clean. She spent most of the day playing cards on the lawn, visiting with the other guests, who, it seemed, knew either Yiddish or Russian. At specified hours we gathered at the dining hall and took our meals sitting at communal tables.

Phil was still young enough to be content to stay near Mom and play with the few other children his age. Once Marty and I had explored the nearby woods, swam in the muddy pond and completed a marathon Ping-Pong tournament that resulted in the inevitable furious fist fight, we became bored and looked for more interesting activities. Basham Lake, ten miles or so away, was where we wanted to go. Mom would not take us. Because we were convinced she would not disturb her card-playing routine to please us it led to a grinding, attritional, although non-confrontational struggle. We knew too well that confronting Mom was not a safe tactic. Instead, we were surly and uncooperative. We whined. We dragged ourselves around. We found fault with everything. The woods, full of cool mysteries days before, became overly humid and full of biting insects. The pond, formerly an exciting vantage point for thirsty deer and water snakes, was now a fetid, foul smelling, stagnant puddle. Ping-Pong was out of the question. The racquets were inferior and the ball had a crack in it. When we grew overbearing Mom snapped at us and gave the occasional slap to assert her authority. Finally, wearied by our tactics, she offered us a bargain. If we behaved until Dad came on the weekend, he would take us to Basham Lake for swimming and rowboating.

Dad arrived late Friday night in a bad temper. The car had been acting up, despite the grudged time away from work arranging repairs, the car still did not run well. It lacked power and sputtered. He was convinced he had been taken advantage of in the original transaction, a pitiless trick played on him, a wrong that could not be righted. He moved with quick, violent energy, his dark face drawn. He said little. We knew he was seething, a dangerous condition. Nevertheless, Marty and I had been promised the trip to Basham Lake. True, not by Dad and we knew well enough that Mom's decisions were always subject to Dad's veto. We pressed ourselves on him, breathlessly telling him of Mom's promise. He glared at her contemptuously and without looking at us, treating our ebullient declaration as a mere inquiry, said to us, dismissively, "We'll see tomorrow." That was enough for us for the moment. We bounded outdoors to take advantage of the remaining minutes of fading daylight.

Dad was still sleeping when we silently left our room, clad in bathing suits. Later, Mom joined us on the lawn and told us conspiratorially that Dad would indeed take us after breakfast; but that we were not to *nudj* him or he would change his mind. Joyfully, we repaired to the bordering woods to wait, reasoning that our absence would guaranty that we would not give offense and risk a change of mind. Every fifteen minutes or so we emerged from the woods to survey the building where our rooms were, the lawn and the dining room. At last, mid-morning, we saw Dad emerge from our quarters and walk to the dining room. As he crossed the lawn, his newspaper under his arm, we could see from our distant vantage point that, even as he greeted people in his path, his face was a grim mask. We waited. He emerged finally, recrossed the lawn and went back to the room to finish his morning ablutions. Marty and I seized the middle ground, the lawn, where we fidgeted until Dad appeared clad in garish bathing trunks with matching shirt, shoes and socks, an armful of towels, polo shirts for us and his newspaper. Mom followed us to the car with a bag of sandwiches and fruit, admonishing us to behave.

Dad did not speak to us on the way to the lake, except to tell us to quiet down. When the car faltered he muttered dark Russian curses under his breath, the ones that made Mom blush. At the lake he lay on one of the towels, his shoes, socks and shirt on, and glued his attention to the newspaper. Marty and I raced to the water, eager to prove to ourselves that we were indeed at Basham Lake. The lake was huge. The opposite shore looked like the horizon.

When we left the water we were chilled and exhausted. Hugging ourselves we tiptoed up the sloped beach. Dad was still reading, a towel over his head for shade.

"Daddy, aren't you going to swim?"

He raised his head, wincing against the sudden stab of sunlight. Looking at us, his skinny, cocoa-brown twin sons, shivering uncontrollably, his face seemed to soften momentarily. "Maybe later. Sit down. Dry yourselves. You should have come out of the water sooner. You'll catch cold like that. Rest and then you'll have a sandwich."

Dad was no longer as dark brown as we were. His skin had yellowed with age. As he shifted position to hand us towels and to uncover the sandwiches we noticed the purple eruptions of varicose veins on his legs. Marty and I dried vigorously and sat carefully on the part of the towel Dad shared with us. We ate our sandwiches quickly, with spare movement, attempting to precisely time the completion of the meal with the return to the water.

"You're not going in the water yet. You'll get cramps. Sit quietly for a while."

"How long?"

Dad looked at us witheringly. "Until I say you can get up." His attention was returning to the newspaper.

"Will you go swimming with us?"

"Yes, yes, when it's time for you to go back in."

Marty and I sat for a minute or two in a state of suppressed excitement. The possibilities for the day were opening. We couldn't just sit and watch Dad, his motionlessness broken only by the rhythmic licking of his thick finger as he turned the page of the newspaper and smartly snapped it open and then shut to isolate the continuation of the article he was reading.

"Daddy, can we walk down the beach? We won't run." Tensing, we waited for the answer.

The hooded eyes turned toward us, the cobra head turning ever so gracefully, but the voice was not annoyed. "Where will you go? When will you be back?"

"Just down the beach to the boat dock. We'll be back in not too long."

Life suspended in that viscous moment between question and answer. He considered.

"All right, but don't run, and be back in a half hour."

We loved watching Dad swim. We were both amused and admiring of the execution of his powerful modified crawl, his mouth pursed, every deliberate stroke seeming to shoot his body half out of the water and fly ahead to a dead stop. A strong swimmer with mighty endurance, he assumed we were too as he swam, unconcerned as to our whereabouts. After a time Marty and I returned to the shallows while Dad continued stroking, resting by floating on his back.

When he rejoined us and his feet touched the ground he straightened, smoothed his thinning, still black hair straight back with both hands and let out a lung-clearing roar. He was smiling. He played with us, throwing us up in the air in turns, where we twisted and squirmed and hit the water with great splashes. We swam between his legs, daring him to imprison us with a scissors hold. When he swam a few strokes in mock flight we attacked him underwater, grabbing his feet and trying to pull him under. As he lost steerage he kicked to right himself and hit my shoulder hard with his toe. He withdrew his foot convulsively and stroked to the shore, hobbling on to the sand, in pain, muttering to himself. The only word we could understand as we followed him back to the towel, spat more than said, was "kids."

"Daddy, it was an accident. I didn't mean it."

"I know, I know. I just want to sit here for a while. Then we'll go back." His face showed the pain.

Marty and I were standing, poised, nervously attentive, surrounding him, looking down at him. Dad's leg was outstretched, his head bent, considering his toe, which he was flexing to test the injury. "But Daddy", we said almost in unison, "we haven't gone out in the boat yet."

Dad lifted his head sharply. Something in our earnest, disappointed, faces, detained him from issuing an unanswerable dictate, a command that would have cast us both into sullen, sorrowful silence. "It's the middle of the afternoon. They probably make you rent the boat at the beginning of the day. If they have any left they probably charge for the whole day anyway."

"No, they have boats. We saw when we went for a walk after lunch. You can rent one for an hour if you want. We asked." We leaned forward, crowding him, our faces hopeful.

He thought. He fished his watch out of his shirt pocket and studied it. He looked beyond us into the sky and then down to the shoreline, surveying, considering.

"Okay, put everything into the car. I'll drive over to the boat dock. If they have a boat we'll go out for an hour or so, no more. It will start getting chilly after that."

We jumped up and down in delight. "Can we row the boat?"

"Yes, yes, but get moving or we won't go at all."

Dad rowed like he swam, with long, slow, powerful strokes, bending into his work with concentration. Within minutes we were begging to row. Dad yielded his seat, gave each of us an oar and instructed us to pull together. The boat made a zigzag course, frustrating us. "How do you row straight when you can't see where you're going?"

"Make sure the wake is straight."

"What's the wake?"

"The bubbles that come out behind the boat. You each have to pull together or you'll go crooked."

Out intention to cooperate foundered after a couple of minutes. We eyed each other furtively, suspecting the other of subtly sabotaging the enterprise by randomly alternating the rhythm of the stroke. Marty's elbow caught me smartly in the ribs. I responded by hitting him with my shoulder hard enough to knock him against the gunwale. Both tensed for combat, we dropped the oars.

"Th-th-that's enough," shouted Dad, "g-g-get in the b-b-b-back right now and sit quietly." The menace of his stutter-contorted face quieted us. We crept to the back of the boat silently, doubly upset because we had frittered away our opportunity by our own stupidity, or more correctly, each of us thought, by the stupidity of the other. Dad installed himself on the middle thwart and began rowing while Marty and I looked out at the water from different sides of the boat, resentfully avoiding the other. At least dad wasn't rowing directly back to the boat dock, summarily ending the day. Maybe he'd let us row later.

Within minutes, the argument flared anew. One thought the other had strayed over the imaginary line dividing the thwart we shared. A shove removing the invader provoked a retaliatory poke; our tinny, changing voices prodding the other with insults erupted finally in a flailing of fists and feet.

"Goddamn it, stop it," roared Dad, "you kids, y-y-you beg to be t-t-taken out here and all you can do is f-f-f-fight." His face was exploding.

"But Daddy," we both started to say in our defense and in condemnation of the other.

"Shut the hell up!"

The battle between Marty and me had passed the point of mediation. Heedless of Dad's wrath, one kicked the other in the leg pushing the other's foot sharply into Dad's injured toe. Dad let out a wounded cry and as he reflexively withdrew his foot he smashed it into the side of the boat. We leaped to our feet. The look on his face, which we had seen only a few times in our life, showed that he was beyond reason. "Get the hell out of the boat!"

We stood dumbly, not wanting to understand. He leaned forward in a crouch and with a sweep of his arm he knocked one of us over the gunwale into the water. The remaining one jumped over the side before he could do the same to him. Dad sat heavily and with one stroke of the oars put distance between us. We paddled madly toward the boat, which was now flying from us. Dad was not even looking at us. With murderous intensity he was abandoning us.

Terrified, we treaded water, watching Dad recede rapidly from our sight. Alone in the water, we were perhaps a quarter mile from the nearest shore in a direction almost opposite from where Dad was headed. Crying and trembling, we began swimming resolutely, measuring our strokes carefully, neither one wanting to inflame the fears of the other. We swam side by side, grateful for the occasional touch of the other. We didn't stop till we reached the shore. Hunkering on the grassy bank, we consoled each other without words, wondering what would happen next, glad to be away from Dad for now.

The sun was lower in the sky and a gentle wind was rising. We were shivering. To arrive at the paved road we stepped gingerly through a field, avoiding rocks, stickers and cow pies. We could see the boat dock around the curve of the lake. That was where Dad would have to come from if he was going to pick us up, if he wasn't going to make us walk all the way back. We smiled at each other, feeling adventurous. At least we hadn't drowned. After a few minutes we turned in the other direction and began walking back to Lena's, chattering to each other with bravado. We felt tough. We wondered where Dad was, but we were not anxious to encounter him.

Arriving at a fork in the road some thirty or forty minutes later, we stood, our shoulders slumping, our spirits sagging, unsure of which road led to Lena's. Exhausted and cold, tears forming, we looked at each other to determine if any there was any reserve of courage left to be shared. The awkward, pudgy Nash Ambassador crunched to a stop on the gravelly shoulder fifty feet ahead. We scuttled toward it and tentatively opened the back door. Dad had turned sideways in his seat and regarded us with an expression we took to be neutral.

"Wipe your feet. If your bathing suits are wet be sure to sit on a towel."

Our feet wiped, we entered and sat on the towel, deep in the seat, close to each other, touching, grateful to be sharing the enclosed space.

Before we turned twelve we graduated from our sixth grade school, prepared to go on to junior high school, were in the midst of studying for our bar mitzvah, and discovered sex, or more correctly, masturbation. Neither the religious nor the academic commitment interfered in the slightest with the obsession that possessed us as well as the dozen or so boys of our age in the neighborhood: to achieve ejaculation. During the two weeks we spent in Boy Scout camp that summer we had a live demonstration provided by one of the older boys. In a clearing in the woods, a goodly walk from the center of the camp, the ten boys or so who were to be instructed in the art of onanism, formed a circle around the teacher.

As he removed his pants and underwear, he slowly talked to us about practicing the solitary art. Lying on a bed of leaf litter, he began stroking his penis, formidable looking to his audience of much younger boys. With awe, tinged with fear at the sight of the forbidden, we listened raptly and watched without blinking as he manipulated himself to an erection, all the while talking about naked women, about breasts and vaginas. His breathing became measured, his stroking, in broken rhythm, more concentrated. The head of his penis was swollen, alert, on the upstroke descending to the top of his fist, on the downstroke plunging skyward. After a time his speech stopped in mid word, his belly began trembling and his hand pistoned at triple time. He groaned as great, milky, viscous globs of semen geysered, shooting a foot in the air. Six or seven times he erupted, his body contracting each time. Gradually, with slow, even stroke, he milked the remaining undischarged semen from his penis and languorously resting his head in the leaves, let his entire body relax. The rest of us, his attentive audience, exhaled in unison for what seemed like the first time since the performance started. It was a powerful demonstration and it inspired all of us to practice until we had mastered the skill.

Each of our group stealthily probed his parents' hiding places searching for salacious material. Marty and I found a crude cartoon, beneath Dad's socks, showing a barnyard in which all the animals had human faces and outsized genitalia and were engaged in what we thought at the time were imaginative sexual poses. It shocked us somewhat to conclude that our father had such degenerate tendencies.

We had a rather sketchy notion of what the great purpose of ejaculating was, even less of how it was to be accomplished without masturbating. Our crude knowledge of female anatomy and the tender feelings young romantics like us had would not let us imagine how this act could be performed mechanically with a woman, or rather, a girl. Despite all the dirty talk we heard on the street we wondered how a girl could permit herself to be dirtied so. What kind of a boy would inflict such an indignity upon the girls we knew? What we did know, not yet through experience but from the oral evidence we considered to be beyond question, was that when we were successful it would feel better than anything we had ever known in our lives.

And so, we practiced. Everything, it seemed was practice. Learning the dates and places of our history class required practice. We went dutifully to our Hebrew classes and listened to the green complected seminary students with wispy beards, who taught us to read and write simple Hebrew. We appeared once a week at the musty study of Mr. Horowitz, the Cantor of the synagogue, who patiently taught us to chant the portion of the sacred writings appropriate to the date of our bar mitzvah. After a week of memorizing the text and the cantellations, we would display the our progress to Mr. Horowitz, who sat and listened, his eyes closed, his head nodding rhythmically, stroking his tobacco stained beard, interrupting only when a mistake was made.

After school, and then later, after Hebrew school and still later, after an hour or two of basketball or touch football, Marty and I went home to dinner. We closed the bathroom door behind us to wash our hands and standing alongside of each other, practiced. We tried alternating the rhythm, the pressure. In quiet voices we spoke our fantasies of escapades with women with big breasts who let us have our way with them, wantons who enjoyed it. Although our erections seemed to increase in size daily, nothing happened, no ejaculation. We watched each other, wondering who would accomplish the great feat first. We tried masturbating the other one. There was no shame, no embarrassment. It was as if handling one's own body. We stayed in the bathroom until Mom called us for dinner, and as we tumbled out toward the kitchen feigning nonchalance, we wondered what variations could be employed that night in bed that might lead to the breakthrough we were desperately awaiting.

At last we succeeded, within a day of the other. We were men. Ejaculating was more a sign of arriving at manhood than bar mitzvah. All the boys who had told us of the joys of "coming," were right. It was glorious. We couldn't wait till we could lock the bathroom door or get into bed at night. We were indefatigable. Pleased with our new found ability we did it whenever we could. Now we would talk with confidence about "beating the meat" or "whacking off." No longer would Mom have to pound on the bathroom door before dinner. We would fly into the bathroom after a strenuous afternoon at the schoolyard, wash our hands, masturbate, and be ready for dinner in about two minutes. Included in the two minutes was an inspection of the wall behind the bathtub to be certain that, in our momentary delirium, our cupped hand had not failed to contain the cannonaded stream of semen. For some time we were too concerned with perfecting our solitary techniques to combine forces, but in time we sought to augment the experience. Occasionally, usually in bed, we spun fantasies that we acted out upon each other's body. Now, in contrast to the pre-ejaculation days, we were always successful. There was never any pattern as to who would play what role. If it was a fantasy in which one would be submissive and one dominant, we would scrupulously alternate roles.

We did not consider these activities to be homosexual. We had heard of "homos," men who were effeminate and who swished around, dressed like women and did things, sexual things, with other men. We believed, as did all our contemporaries, that such behavior was disgusting. Marty and I never thought we were doing anything disgusting. We thought only of having sex with girls one day, not with boys. But between Marty and me, there was little difference whether one did things to the body of the other or had things done to his body by the other. It was a form of masturbation with many exquisite variations. We simply had two bodies that could be combined imaginatively. We knew precisely what the other was feeling when stimulated by a touch, by hearing an idea, by seeing a picture. There was no approximation or guess about the others' experience. It was exact, beyond discussion. We didn't make the distinction between Marty's body and mine. We didn't know where one body ended the other began.

In Junior High School, we intensified our cultivation of separate interests with friends not shared by the other, friends who saw only one person, not an identical pair, friends who responded to the characteristics of only one person, friends who said they had no difficulty in telling us apart. Marty studied French and I studied Latin.

Walking the mile or so home, Marty and I attached to different groups. As we strolled each of us saw the other with friends and classmates, chatting, exhibiting mannerisms foreign to the other. Both of us were outraged by the disloyal behavior of the other. It was probably the first time we could see the other twin interact with others, as a singleton. Seeing that it was possible to be treated as an individual and not as a part of a twin strengthened our resolve to differentiate one from the other. Our rivalry intensified.

We were the exact physical and intellectual equal of the other. Both good athletes, if we competed against each other, one on one, the margin of victory was always so slight that the argument following the contest almost always ended in a fight. It was a confusing and frightening time for us. Alternating between a loathing for the other, expressed in physical violence, and the love we felt for each other, sometimes sexually expressed, we both longed to be away from the other without being able to imagine how we could survive apart. There were times when, within a few days we would beat each other until we ached, crawl into one bed for a time, sexually pleasure each other, and, usually of a Saturday morning, read Kipling's epic poems aloud to each other, competing to see who could memorize more of the Barrack Room Ballads or the Ballad of Boh Da Thone or the Ballad of East and West.

Going to different high schools was the greatest physical separation Marty and I had ever experienced. He traveled by subway to Manhattan every day to Stuyvesant High School, an all boys school of students precociously interested in math and science. I went to the nearest high school, Erasmus Hall. For the first time in our lives, at the age of fourteen, we saw the world, a slightly larger world than we had ever known before, through different eyes.

Going to different schools was the beginning of the final break of our shared environment. After all these years I don't remember it as either traumatic or liberating. We didn't plan it or discuss the change nor did we analyze it or appraise it while it was happening. It just happened because it had to. It was like watching high clouds, boldly etched against a brilliant sky. The shapes they assume appear solid at first, sculpted from white marble, immutable. Shortly, they begin to change. The edges soften. Slowly, they reform. The eye quickly accommodates to the shift. Each change is recorded only momentarily. In minutes, the cloud is different or gone, blown away by the stratospheric winds. All that is left is surprise and sketchy memory.

We each absorbed ourselves in what was becoming our separate ways, pursuing activities and interests that the other one did not share. Although we differentiated ourselves in the outside world, we saw each other daily at home and settled into the identity we shared, monitoring and evaluating the changes. We could look at the other, the mirror, and determine whether the pace and direction of the changes was appropriate, whether one could emulate the other, whether one could survive without the other.

At Stuyvesant Marty was surrounded by boys from all over New York City who ran wild with enthusiasm for math and science. His math was much more advanced than the courses I took, which were in fulfillment only of the basic requirements. I struggled to pass. Marty excelled at it. He brought home stories about his new friends, boys who played chess seriously, boys who belonged to after school math and science clubs, boys who plotted mental graphs composed of statistical compilations of the frequency of their masturbations. It was there that Marty discovered the excitement of the mind and developed the diligence to successfully plod through course work. Marty did well in high school. I was an average student.

When we did part, at seventeen, there was no ceremony, no expressed regrets. We simply drifted away, carrying some of the other deeply hidden within. Until we came into contact again. Then all the old, submerged, feelings and behavior would reappear, the secure, cublike, feelings as well as the competitiveness. Over decades of separation, except for sporadic visits and communications, we learned to temper both parts of the ancient feelings. A slight formality recognized that separation, replacing the twinness, that intimacy with the interior of the other. What remained was the shadow of the ache of our loss. We refined the competitiveness until it became a parlor joke, usually taking care not to do injury to the feelings of the other.

Marty's higher education began at City College in New York City. He worked at various menial jobs while he went to school, as much to earn money as to assert his independence from our parents. His performance was lackluster. Working as a clerk and rackpusher in the garment district, developing a social life, and, generally, trying to figure out what to do with his life, drained him of energy for study.

Accepted at the last minute, I went to the University of Vermont. Unable to concentrate on my studies, I devoted myself to learning how to drink and play poker, and made periodic visits to the whorehouses in Montreal, a hundred miles away. I flunked all my courses. They asked me to leave. I returned to New York where I enrolled in City College and repeated the Vermont performance. I didn't last the full semester.

Around this time, seemingly independent of the other, both Marty and I developed an interest in Mexico and Latin America. I can't explain it. Perhaps the great wave of migration from the Caribbean to New York occurring at that time had something to do with it. Perhaps, beneath our consciousness we knew it could be a subject of common interest that could assist us in maintaining the thread of a relationship if all else failed or maintaining a subject of rivalry. Perhaps, though, it is as simple and as inexplicable as being twins. That interest remained with both of us for life. Marty became a professional in the field, a Latin Americanist. I have an avid interest to this day.

Within the next year Marty and I sailed on two Scandinavian merchant ships each. A mutual friend had done it the summer before and had told us stories of his voyage. Marty sailed to Jamaica and Venezuela. I went to the Dominican Republic, Honduras and Guatemala. During overlapping periods between ships, Marty and I swapped stories of our adventures: the initial seasickness, the storms, the drunken fights, the port whores, the glimpse of a brutish life that we both knew was not for us. It didn't matter whether it was Angela at the Miramar in La Ceiba or Marisela at Campo Alegre in Venezuela. It didn't matter whether it was a fight with

29

Bjorn that left a disfigured finger or a scalp wound at the hand of Erik. We both saw the flying fish and schools of dolphin and coastal fog and breathed in the full first odor of the tropics as the ship pulled out of sight of the Port Antonio lighthouse heading south. We both learned a bawdy Scandinavian song and memorized the words to the most popular song of the time in the Caribbean, *Piel Canela*. It was the first real experience we each had had with the Spanish speaking tropics and we loved it. Although we had sailed to different places under somewhat different circumstances, we could savor the experience of the other exactly. We had each done exactly the same thing.

I left the ship in New Orleans and, with two other sailors, a Dane and a Norwegian, drifted to California, where I knew I would stay as soon as I saw it. I was not yet nineteen.

Marty resumed school after he returned from sea. The result was the same as before he left. His work was average, his interest low. Undecided about the future, he went into the army for two years.

In California I worked in factories, machine shops, as a laborer, as a psychiatric technician in a state mental hospital. I took courses sporadically and read constantly. Everything was new and exciting. I went to Mexico twice, for about three months each time. Once, as crew on a sailboat, cruising the western coast. The second time, with friends, where we established ourselves in Guadalajara. I wanted to be a writer, I told myself. I wrote in random bursts, without discipline, without learning how to do it. My life proceeded without plan, without meaningful attachments, without certain trajectory. When I returned to New York from Mexico, broke, I sought Arline, who I had met the year before. Then my path was certain. We married when she was twenty and I less than a year older.

Eight months after we were married and Arline four months pregnant, we left New York for California. With our savings of about six hundred dollars and all our belongings in a used station wagon, we set off for our new life together. I told Arline that I wanted to write but that she should expect the material life that the wages of a skilled factory worker could provide. In her wisdom she didn't question my silly and bravado declaration. Those were the years of the Eisenhower prosperity, the mid to late fifties, and jobs were plentiful. We were young and in love and full of the optimism and courage that love reinforces.

In southern Utah Arline fainted in the western sun and began to bleed. I was terrified. An old doctor in St. George said that she appeared strong, but couldn't predict whether she'd lose the baby and that if it were he, he'd get to California as soon as possible. We rested for a day and drove straight through to our waiting friends who lived south of Los Angeles. The aircraft industry was booming. Several days after we arrived in California I had a job running a turret lathe in a production machine shop.

Marty's two years were up and with his G.I. Bill he enrolled at U.C.L.A., where he finished his Bachelor's. While an undergraduate he took classes in anthropology and traveled to Mexico several times. It interested him as nothing had before. Over the next six years he studied Spanish, for which he showed a great affinity, completed his doctorate and assisted in field work in the valley of Oaxaca. For his widely praised Masters thesis he did field work among the Chocó, a people living in a tropical rain forest in northern Colombia. He lived for several months along the bank of a river that rose and fell five feet in a single day in a region that received 250 inches of rain a year. He knew beyond a doubt both that he wanted to be a cultural anthropologist and that his interest lay more in the field than in the classroom.

Arline and I rented a house, a large, flimsy cottage owned by a courtesan of a bygone Hollywood era. The house, on the beach near Malibu, rented for the princely sum of seventy- five dollars a month. Marty moved in with us, paying twenty dollars a month out of his G.I. Bill allotment of one hundred ten dollars a month, to help us to afford it.

It was odd living with Marty. We hadn't lived together for perhaps five years. By now conscious of the harmful, or at least unpleasant, aspects of twin rivalry, we discussed openly how we would conduct ourselves, made general rules for getting along. After all, our lives were considerably different now. Marty was a student, free of any but self-imposed obligations. I was a married man with responsibilities. We talked of how the house would be run, schedules, and duties. I worked the swing shift at an aircraft factory an hour away and didn't return till one in the morning. I appreciated that Arline would not be alone during most evenings. Marty would be there, attentive and protective toward her.

It was a good arrangement and yet, something about it that I couldn't define was vaguely troubling. Perhaps it was that, because our lives had diverged, we each had both privileges and drawbacks that the other didn't. I had the connubial pleasures of being married, but also the obligation to care for Arline and our baby to come. Without a college degree or a developed trade my prospects were limited, although in that time of plenty, I was confident. Marty had his freedom. He was accountable to no one. He had the time and the circumstance to be deliberate in deciding what

31

to do with his life. All his options were open. Our lives had different characteristics, ones that the other could either envy or feel superior to. It was the first time in our lives that was true.

One night Arline and I returned to the house to find Marty crouched on the couch. He told us, almost apologetically, that a splinter flew into his eye as he had broken a piece of kindling. He couldn't remove it and, in pain, waited some hours for us to get home. The affected eye was the good one, the eye not damaged in the childhood accident. The prospects were fearsome. If this accident rendered Marty's good eye unusable he would virtually be blind. A blind student, a blind anthropologist? How could he continue to travel to Mexico, to the field? We touched on these questions as I drove him the thirty miles to the hospital in Santa Monica. There they removed the deeply imbedded splinter. It had superficially scratched his iris. For a few days he saw the scratch and, although it vanished without leaving any permanent damage the incident left us both shaken.

It reminded us both of the power each of us had to strongly affect the other, whether we consciously tried to exercise it or not. There was nothing we could do about it. We couldn't turn it off. We were still too close. I don't remember if we saw it that way at the time or, if we did, whether we would have had the courage to separate yet again voluntarily. We didn't have to decide. Within weeks of Marty's eye accident a brush fire, with our house at its center, burned some seventy thousand acres and two hundred houses. While our house didn't burn, the area was too devastated to return to. Arline and I were taken in by my cousin in west Los Angeles. We were refugees, awaiting the birth of our baby.

Marty found temporary quarters with a friend and shortly moved into a place of his own. In about a year Arline and I and our year old son, Jonathan, moved to Arizona. It was the last time Marty and I lived in the same city. From the time we graduated from high school, with the exception of that period of a few months, we never lived together again. We formed families, exulted in the birth of children, increased the skill in our different work through success and failure. We lived. We formed different views of the world, of politics, of family and child rearing, of society. We became different people outwardly, we became individuals. Apart. Singletons. Almost completely.

We were aware of the other's progress through sporadic visits, family news, even an occasional exchange of letters. The contact between us was neither intense nor frequent and that suited us. We were forming ourselves as adults in almost completely different environments. During that time I could not be quite sure of what Marty was thinking about the world, about earning a living, about marriage and children, about Vietnam, about me.

There were things about his life that I envied, I was proud of, I resented. He was a researcher in an exciting field, teaching in a prestigious school, the holder of a doctorate. He traveled to places I longed to see, but believed I never would. I was a struggling small businessman in the Southwest without even a bachelor's degree. He was in an insulated world, I told myself, his tenured position was a sinecure, and he and all the people of his acquaintance agreed with each other. They all knew that they were right and people like me, struggling to make a living selling real estate, were all wrong. Martin once told me, when, I presumed he was involved in a Marxist study group, that, as a broker, I belonged to the non-productive element of society. It hurt me at the time. It took me many years to realize that, in the Marxist sense, he belonged to the same group. I felt I was closer to the daily experience of ordinary people than he was and that gave me a better credential for understanding society. I considered, with a certain pride, that I lived in a hostile world, doing battle against philistines who forced me to defend myself in business and in my social and political values. People in my cutthroat environment would try to take my livelihood from me and were constantly condemning my beliefs as being too liberal. I was always in the minority. In my private thoughts I melodramatically overstated our differences. I drew comfort in feeling sorry for myself. I also felt proud, however, that my views, being somewhere between what I believed to be the northeastern academic, insular, rote leftism and the anti-analytical southwestern country conservatism, were balanced, freeing me to criticize and to draw from both ideological poles.

I was doing poorly at my trade, barely supporting my family, which now included three children. My work gave me no enjoyment and I secretly despaired of ever being good enough at it to be prosperous. My earning uncertainty was wearing on Arline, creating tension between us. At times I longed for a civil service job, anything to remove the economic cloud we seemed to be living under.

Marty's career was thriving. His reputation was spreading. He was doing work he was passionately interested in, work that was deemed by the world to be important. Between his ever increasing salary and grants for research and travel, he was living much better than I was. I was jealous of Marty and I was ashamed of my feelings.

The worst of it was that I ceased to be sure of what Marty was thinking of me. The days of having the anticipatory knowledge of what Marty was thinking that I had as a child were gone. Without being able to articulate it, or perhaps being too frightened to, I felt the loss of what we once had and that I believed could never be recaptured.

THE NEWS

Oct. 31, 1971
Dear Saul,

It was very good to speak to you Friday night. It was also very painful since within the last two weeks my life has taken an abrupt and difficult turn. During my routine health checkup, I was told that I'm suffering from a form of leukemia. My disease, chronic lymphocytic leukemia, showed up in a blood test in a form of significant imbalance of white blood cells with an abnormal concentration of one kind (lymphocytes). I have no other symptoms now and felt fine all this past year. This disease eventually causes anemia that in turn creates susceptibility to other symptoms and disorders, and finally death. It is at present incurable, although there are medications that can ease symptoms and restore the balance of blood cell production. Between outbreaks of symptoms that may require medication and hospitalization, patients can live fairly normal lives. While it is hard to get any clear idea of my life expectancy from this point (doctor's don't really know, and the crude level of euphemism makes all their speech sound hollow), judging from the rate of increase in white blood count from two years ago when I had my last test, I am given to understand that I should think of the future in terms of years. I've been told that people have lived twenty years like this without medication. That was told to me as a figure that <u>might occur so I think a more cool estimate would reduce that.</u>

Since getting this news, I've been living a hell that I never believed could hurt so much. For the first week, Wilma and I cried our eyes out. During this time, we managed to carry on most of our activities and movements. In fact, we are moving toward "normalizing" our life; at least feeling the urge to break down less and less. Wilma's love and understanding are a powerful help to me, and in that painful bittersweet way, make for an intensity and depth of experience and feeling that only an adversity like this can produce. I know that once I pull through this first awful shock, life will be a very different proposition and, hopefully, maybe because of it, can provide some satisfactions and meaning.

For now, I'm hurting. I feel scared constantly. In my stomach and in acid sweat that seems to boil out of me my main feelings are anxiety (fear, tension) and depression. I conjure all the horrors that have been formed by a lifetime of listening to tragedies that happen to others in books, conversations and through observation. Right now, everything I hear or see has an interpretation for me that only bodes death. Quiet moments are the hardest. Before sleeping and waking I'm tortured by explicit scenes of how my end will come, what I'll say, feel like, look like plus all the other particulars that are associated with it. When I do some commonplace thing around the house, with it's implication of stability and continuity, with all the built-in understandings of time to come, time to make it right, time to improve, I feel my strength leak away—I feel weak, winding down, dying. Holding Aaron, for whom we waited so long, gives me such sadness as well as the sense that I still have the right and the duty of fathering him and his sister. I think of my family, the kids, our moment, our reality.

Saul, I write to you because I can't do otherwise. One of my first thoughts when I was told about this was of us starting out together, our bond, and now the fact of an end. I was fearful of telling you, maybe that you would see this as the ultimate rank and be angry. It's really beyond that now. I see that holding back is much more painful than confronting it. You are the first person I've told after Wilma and I think in time I will include more people as I learn to see myself in this new reality. For now it seems too hard to tell the folks. I don't mean to exclude Arline but this is a letter to you that you can share with her if you wish. I'm in constant flux, talking to Wilma a lot and with the help of analysis. I'll stay in touch and share my thoughts.

Marty

I had no suspicion of his being ill until the moment I read his letter. He and Wilma had a six year old daughter, Leah, and just had their second child after a guarded pregnancy. A child that had died just after birth and an earlier miscarriage had made the arrival of Aaron all the sweeter. Marty was 36 years old and leading an energetic life, actively tending his career and his family, planning field trips, planning vacations, believing in a limitless future, planning, always planning. Suddenly, it all seemed out of reach. Leukemia had ruined it all.

His letter to me would have seemed strange to most people. It described the confirmation of this terrible illness as "abrupt and difficult." He was understating it to spare me. And to spare him the added pain that he would feel in direct proportion to the anguish and sorrow I would feel. He asked me to understand that he was not trying to outdo me or "one-up" me, to overpower me with the terrible news. In the street talk of the Brooklyn of the 1940's and early 50's he was not "ranking" me.

I read the letter several times, put it carefully in my pocket so that nobody could learn my secret and left my small and crowded office in Phoenix so that no one would see me cry. I walked around the streets for an hour or so crying and snuffling, unable to clarify my thoughts. All I knew in that moment was that my brother, my twin brother, that part of me that I knew would always be there with me, was leaving, was tearing something loose from my body, from my mind, from my existence. If he died, it was the end of me. I was bereft.

Immediately after the diagnosis, Arline and I began reading about leukemia. We went to the public library, looked up articles on the subject and tried to read them. It was difficult and frustrating. I discovered quickly how important information was to me as a talismanic source of assurance. I believed I would be calmed by letting knowing take the place of imagining. Even if the information led to the conclusion that the worst had to be faced - Martin's early death - I believed it would strengthen me to know precisely what I would have to face. Most of the information was impenetrable. I didn't want the long course in hematology, histology and immunology. I didn't want to have to learn a new language to understand the rudiments of my brother's disease. I wanted conclusions, true and concise.

The closest I came was in several conversations I had with doctors who had written articles on the subject. In each case the doctors were straightforward. They could hear the distress in my voice as I tried to ask the questions I so desperately needed answered. They responded clearly, with business-like detachment and volunteered information I hadn't known enough to ask for. They let me know in their kind inflection that they knew how it hard it was for us all. I was grateful for their treatment. They each refused payment.

I put together a file of what I had learned. I thought about it. It did calm me and I knew it would calm Marty. The understanding I had gained was that Martin's disease was usually a slowly progressing one and that more than half of the sufferers of chronic lymphocytic leukemia live for more than five years after they are diagnosed. Medical statistics are bewildering to lay people. They relate, as they must, to large groups of people, thought to share the same disease. The problem is that each case has sufficient individual variations so that the sufferer can't possibly tell with what force the statistic affects his case. This five year statistic sounded to me initially like *farthings per furlong per fortnight*. Still, it gave me a certain degree of comfort. Martin was not in danger of dying soon. The very term chronic, instead of acute, had a softer ring. It also seemed clear that many patients have the disease for years before they are diagnosed and some have the disease, are never diagnosed, and live out their normal life span.

I knew I had to talk to Marty and Wilma, face to face.

I met Marty in New York City in the spring of 1972. He was attending a meeting of the American Anthropological Association, the "triple A", he and his colleagues called it. The plan was to spend the last day or two of the convention with him and travel together back to Boston. I hadn't seen him in some time, perhaps two years. I met him in the hotel lobby before I checked in. He was watching me approach when I noticed him, his face shining with a cracked, open smile. The smile was partly in mischievous delight at the shock I would register when I saw him unexpectedly and partly at the pleasure of being together after all this time, without extended family, just he and I. And hundreds of milling anthropologists. I dropped my bag as he approached. We shook hands strongly, pumping, squeezing, edging closer to each other. We slapped the others' shoulder. Finally, Marty put his arms around me. I followed his example and we briefly banged each others backs with palms. Because of his time in Mexico he was accustomed to giving and receiving *abrazos*. I was not.

"How are you?"

"Fine. How are you?"

"Fine." We both laughed at the nervous aridity of the greeting. His eyes held mine, conveying a shy longing. After all these years of physical separation we were both signalling that even in this first instant we had refreshed the same complete understanding of the other we had had as children. Almost. A tiny, metallic light in the eye, a defensive beacon, said, "almost". The final step would be here soon though, and we were both pleased and relieved that the other was exactly as remembered.

"This is not a great place to talk," said Marty. His expression tightened, reminding me that his colleagues surrounding us knew nothing of his illness.

I searched him with my eyes for changes. I detected none. He was the same Martin, my same Marty. Hair black, eyes brown, complexion olive. About five ten. Lean and quick of movement, with inquisitive, moving eyes. He radiated vitality.

How stupid I felt. What on earth did I expect? Did I think that I could look through his skin, into his arteries and veins and see those cancer damaged leukocytes swimming around with malevolent expressions? Could I see his cells becoming cancerous and growing wildly, crowding out the normal ones? And yet, Marty had cancer of the blood-forming tissues. When you have cancer you are supposed to be very sick. Marty did not look sick at all.

How many times over the next twenty-odd years would I hear people say how well Marty looked or sounded, people who knew for a certain fact that he had leukemia? How false and stupid and cowardly I thought it sounded in the beginning. I took their reaction to mean that they would say anything to avoid facing the horrible truth of the possibility of death. Since then my attitude has tempered a great deal. I realize now that because there is no correct or satisfying response to the awful news of the disease or impending death of a friend or a loved one, most people who hear this news freeze. They immediately, either consciously or instinctively, determine which role they believe to be the correct one, for both themselves and the sufferer. News such as this is so ugly and so rare that people are unable to know what they are feeling and, in their search for safety in the moment, repair to reactions that are mannered. And then, more often than not, denial follows.

"Are you sure of the diagnosis?"

"They are making great advances in this disease."

"My uncle Louie has had the same thing for the last 43 years. He still looks great."

"You'll lick it. You're made of strong stuff."

"I forgot where the article appeared, but it was about someone with the same disease who saw this healer in the mountains of Borneo who cured him in no time."

"I can't believe it."

One friend of his at the time, an economist, suggested to him with ponderous, professorial seriousness, that he discuss his inheritance, if any, with our parents. After all, if he was going to die soon anyway, why not enjoy his last?

The truth is that no reaction is good or entirely appropriate. Even letting the heart speak without censor may not be the best thing for those involved. When Marty and Wilma experienced the death of their baby after 36 hours of life, I asked what we could do for them in their grief. Marty told me that there was nothing that anyone could do for them except to cry with them. It is true. All anyone can do to assist another in their grief is to sit, mute and dazed, like the young parents I saw in Nicaragua, many years later, staring at their dead infant daughter, a white sprig in her mouth, cheeks rouged, while a weathered relative sawed the boards outside their hut for the small coffin. I have sympathy now for those who hear about Marty for the first time. It's hard for them. For all of us, Marty's family, for those who love him, it is hard. It is now and it always will be.

One of the speakers at the meeting was Carlos Castaneda, Marty's fellow graduate student at U.C.L.A. who had achieved a great deal of fame for his books about Don Juan, a northern Mexican wise man/sorcerer. Carlos' work had begun with an investigation of the effects of certain psychotropic drugs, a subject of intense interest to the young scholars, one felt an interest not entirely academic. The large lobby in the hotel, choked with anthropologists, was abuzz with anticipation of Carlos's arrival.

The standard dress of the attendees was rags, clothing that was loose fitting, with obvious signs of overwear. The accouterment to the dress, however, was a huge quantity of ethnic art, accessories and jewelry. A mountain of turquoise, a warehouse of feathers, hats of every description, bracelets, sandals, amulets, talismans floated by in a display that looked to my eye like a museum exhibit gathered from the remote places of the world. Martin and I walked through the cavernous lobby together.

I observed with great interest all that was going on. It fascinated me that just outside the hotel people were marching up and down the busy midtown Manhattan street, near the garment center, dressed in business suits and ties, hurrying to their commercial rounds. Some were hourly workers, office workers on break, rack pushers on their way to a delivery; others were the ubiquitous big city wanderers, like stage props, being dragged along by the energy of the human current entrapping them. People who were selling things, buying things, trying to outthink their commercial adversaries, trying to do deals, trying to advance themselves in a way that could be reckoned in money. I understood them. Although my daily activities were different from theirs I understood their motives, their drive. I felt a certain kinship with them, and born of that kinship was sympathy for them.

Inside it was different. The huge public space was densely packed and wildly animated. I imagined that if seen from thirty feet above, the people below would resemble microorganisms seen through a microscope. A small group would agitate with conversation and arm movements and body gestures only to reform itself into a different size to accommodate a member added or subtracted. Arms penetrated like jungle vines, touching someone walking by or holding someone still to insure the acknowledgment of a greeting offered. The movement was constant. It became apparent shortly, however, that the people in that room were working. Despite the language of friendship, inquiring about each other's families, asking questions that seemed personal, pledging later meetings, it was clear that business was being conducted. From the bits of conversation I heard as I floated through the room, the principal topics were job opportunities, grant sources for field research and publishing possibilities.

Marty and I decided to leave the hotel to have lunch when a corridor seemed to appear in the middle of the crowd and from it, to an audible murmur of respect, stepped Carlos Castaneda. Martin and Carlos embraced. Martin introduced me. We shook hands. A circle of young academics watched Carlos carefully as if willing him to gaze in their direction. In contrast to the garb of the room, Carlos was wearing an expensive-looking gray striped suit with vest and tie. A squat, brown man, his black hair was short and neatly combed. Apparently, to counter the attractiveness of drug use many young people felt his work portrayed, he comported himself in as straightlaced and uncool a way as possible.

Marty invited Carlos to join us for lunch and he eagerly accepted. We went to a nearby fish restaurant, a noisy, bustling place with the frequent crash of plates slammed on marble table tops. Marty and Carlos talked. I had read the one or two books he had published at that time and I was more than content to listen. Before the talk of Carlos's work began, Marty asked me surreptitiously if I would mind if he spoke to Carlos in Spanish. He wanted to tell Carlos about his disease, a subject still foreign to him, and it seemed more appropriate to address him in his native Spanish. There was another reason for telling Carlos, with whom Marty had not maintained particularly close relations after graduate school. It was a reason that I agreed with and it described perfectly the fear we both felt at contemplating the onset of Martin's life-threatening disease. Although nobody knew much about his day-to-day life, it was believed that Carlos lived in a world inhabited by sorcerers, witches, herbalists, people of magic. Because he was a trained anthropologist he wrote about these things as a social scientist, but at the same time it seemed clear that he believed them. Somehow, at the time, he appeared to be connected to a world outside that of traditional solutions, of traditional medicine, a world in which the unexpected could happen and did happen.

Martin, and I, had just been told of his leukemia, his cancer. Cancer meant death, leukemia meant death. Despite the research I had done, despite the mortality statistics and all the rest, the doctors were not saying that they knew how to cure this disease. They were saying, in effect, that they did not know how to cure this disease.

They said instead, that if you had to have leukemia, chronic lymphocytic leukemia was the best kind to have and that the Boston area was the best place to have it, that if a bone marrow transplant was ever needed, it was best to have an identical twin. They said that the progress of the disease varies from person to person and that there is no telling when, if ever, it will break out of its relatively benign form. For the time being a conservative therapeutic approach was to be used. Everything the doctors said about the disease was intended to build confidence, to alleviate worry, to be as cheery as possible. Instead, it made the conclusion inescapable that they had no cure.

It was not as if either one of us expected that Carlos would be able to address Martin's leukemia directly by offering something concrete. But perhaps this friend of Don Juan, this acquaintance of Don Genaro, this explorer of the cruel, arid lands of northern Mexico, where magical herbs grow, where *diableros* and *brujos* live, where Indians run hundreds of miles in search of mind-altering drugs, could give Marty a clue, rational or religious, of a cure.

Carlos's reaction to Marty's revelation was abrupt and matter of-fact. "It's nothing," he said, first in Spanish, then in English. "It's shit, Martin. You shouldn't worry about it. I knew someone who had it. He fixed it up in no time. I'll send you something to take for it. Don't worry." He described an herb that both Marty and I thought was angelica. I later looked it up in several reference works. In none of those was there any mention of properties having to do with curing blood diseases or cancers.

The rest of the lunch was devoted to Carlos's work. He told us that his "world had turned." I took it to mean that he no longer felt any obligation to explain one world to the other. Until that time he would explain to his readers what Don Juan meant when he said something alien to our understanding or what really happened when Carlos "experienced" something out of the realm of ordinary experience, like flying. It portended the description of events and experiences presented reportorially in his writing rather than the careful, doubting presentation of the social scientist. He would tell us what happened to him. What part of it was metaphor, what part verifiable reality, the reader would have to decide.

Carlos told us about conversations he had with animals in the northern Mexican desert. He said that he talked to a dung beetle and a coyote. He said that the coyote, in a squeaky, high pitched voice, spoke Spanish like a *pocho*, using English words from time to time. The coyote seemed to be interested in his books. He asked Carlos questions about how the books were selling. The conversation continued in that vein until the end of the lunch. Carlos told us that, as a result of his training with Don Juan, his understanding of the external world was changing and that new experiences were assimilable.

I was excited listening to Carlos. I was an admirer of his work and it was thrilling to me to be able to hear him. Marty, because he was both an old friend and colleague, reacted differently. It seemed to me that he was used to hearing this kind of narrative and, filtering it through his training, he searched for its meaning. The lunch ended and we said good-bye. I felt uplifted for the moment by the possibility, however remote, that Carlos would indeed be instrumental in Marty's cure.

Although Marty had some sporadic contact with him in the next few years, the subject of Martin's leukemia was not discussed, nor did Carlos ever send him any curative herbs.

The rest of our time, another day or so, in New York, passed quickly. I accompanied Marty in his visiting with colleagues, being introduced to his professional society, sitting in on discussions of papers given. We didn't have much time to talk quietly about the reason for my trip. It suited us both. This was the first time I had seen Martin since his diagnosis was confirmed and we were both getting used to dealing with each other in the light of this new, awful knowledge. Simply spending a couple of days in close proximity was a good beginning. We decided to take the train back to Boston.

The journey was one we both tried to infuse with a sentimental nostalgia. We discussed having a resplendent breakfast in the elaborate dining room, being served by elderly, black, uniformed career porters. We imagined sitting in plush seats, alone in a large car, feasting with silver utensils on a white tablecloth, talking softly to each other while watching the New England shore, woodlands and settlements of colonial houses pass swiftly outside the window. We still both smoked in those days. Perhaps a cigar after breakfast to lend proper atmosphere to our conversation about Martin's disease. We would say things to each other, important and profound, that we would remember forever, framed by the wonderful scene we had conjured. The reality, naturally, was something quite different. The eggs were like concrete, the silverware dirty, the tablecloth non-existent and, in general, the train itself, unclean and shabby.

That trip is fixed in my memory. The light, when it burst through the leaden clouds, was harsh as it reflected upon the water or stabbed through the forests of leafless trees. That light, the color of thunder, made each scene viewed through the speeding train window frame seem unique, individual. The junkyards, the piles of abandoned machinery, the dilapidated houses, the pools of stagnant water and chemicals all seemed impersonal, without life, without character, simply a frame for memory. We sat and smoked our cigars, saying little, thinking of the awful thing that reunited us.

The real difficulty was in trying to talk to each other about what had brought us together - the possibility, the probability, or one day the fact, of Marty's death. To be sure, neither one of us had the knowledge or the vocabulary to be able to ask the proper questions about the future and, more importantly, were too stunned by the horror of recent events to be able to speak our hearts to each other. Many years have passed since that subdued train ride from New York to Boston during which time we learned how to talk to each other honestly, through the anger, through the terror, not just about Martin's disease but also about the end of the twins.

Marty and Wilma lived in a large apartment, on the top floor of an old frame house in a working class neighborhood near M.I.T. The old wooden floors creaked, paint was peeled in places. When the spring breezes blew through the open windows and the light penetrated the innards of their apartment, it gave one the warm and confident feeling of childhood, of the secret, consoling holes and hiding places in the apartments in which we were raised. When the wind whipped off the Charles River in the winter and the skies turned to steel gray and black, the inside of the apartment felt gloomy and inhospitable. I had lived by then long enough in the Southwest to need the nourishment of warmth and bright skies.

At a certain moment during my stay with them, I asked them, rather formally and with a nervous flourish, to sit down and hear the result of the research that Arline and I had done. It was somewhat awkward. They politely agreed. I had a file folder full of notes and some zeroxed articles. I tried to be as declarative and matter-of-fact as possible, as if I were presenting them with mildly interesting pieces of information about someone we were barely acquainted with. I was determined to recite the information I had brought and not lecture to Martin, the professional lecturer. They were both determined to appreciate what I was going to say and be grateful to me for it.

It came off well. Most of the information I presented to them, although expressed differently, was well known to them. Some of it was not particularly interesting to them. Some of it, particularly the accounts of the phone conversations I had with leukemia specialists, was both new and of great interest. The opinion that was forming in my mind, when I could calm my imagination, was that it was possible that Martin could live a normal life expectancy. After all, he looked well.

After the diagnosis had settled into all our minds we increased the frequency of our contacts. We called each other more often, we even wrote a little. Our families shared vacation visits several times during the seventies, at the seashore in Massachussetts and twice in southern Mexico where Marty had gone with Wilma and their children for two years to conduct an ethnographic study in a Zapotec speaking village. On one of those visits we stayed close to the city of Oaxaca, making day trips to villages and ruins. During the other we toured the Mayan ruins of Yucatan, Tabasco and Quintana Roo. I had studied Mayan culture and archeology for several years before the trip and seeing some of the ruins for the first time felt like coming home. I felt proud of being able to discuss the sites knowledgeably with Marty.

There I was able to see Marty at work in the environment he loved. I saw him with the villagers he was studying. I sat in on a couple of interviews. I met his native informant a number of times and listened to the questions and answers between them. I attended the patron saint *fiesta*, the most important of the year, as Marty explained to me the significance of all that was happening. He told me, over a period of days, the conclusions he was making about the society he was studying.

He believed that the round of ritual celebrations, the majority of which took place in the fall, after the corn harvest, was a mechanism to redistribute wealth. Different people were selected each year to be the head, or *mayordomo* of the various important *fiestas*. Choosing them was complicated. There was no election. People of influence suggested who might be the *mayordomo*. The person selected could not openly solicit the office, nor could he honorably refuse it. That person was usually someone whose fortunes had been good the recent past years: his crops were in surplus, he had accumulated more land and he had more than enough animals, especially a yoke of oxen. To properly fulfill the task, which involved providing food, drink and entertainment for all in the village for several days, he might have to impoverish himself. All those invited could eat as much as they wanted and could carry food home with them. For those whose crops had not been successful, the extra food gleaned from the *fiestas* over a two month period, made an important difference. The recipients of these needed rations did not have to act as if they were receiving charity. In the future it might be their turn at *mayordomia* and the *mayordomo* of a past *fiesta* might be their guest.

I found Marty's work exciting. I admired greatly the way he comported himself in the village: the way he gathered data, his interviews of villagers over a long period of time and just the way he interacted with both the people he had become familiar with and those with whom he had more formal relations. He belonged there. It was obvious that he respected his subjects. I was thrilled to accompany Marty. It was as if I was doing field work studying an anthropologist doing field work.

With pride, Marty and Wilma guided Arline and me through the countryside, explaining the dress, the foods, the handicrafts, the markets convened the same day of the week continuously for four hundred years, the catholic churches built on the ruins of the Zapotec and Mixtec temples, the colonial heart of the city of Oaxaca, and above all, the social structure of San Sebastian Teitipac, the village he was studying.

Marty, Wilma, and their Mexican friends and colleagues constantly discussed national politics, which had grown turbulent since the government killing of the students at Tlatelolco in 1968. They were fiercely critical of the Mexican government, considering it, among its other failings, to be criminally insensitive to the indigenous. It was 1974 and one of the two years Marty spent in Mexico was his first sabbatical. Three years after the diagnosis of his disease he was engaged, competent and very much alive, his interest extending far beyond the classroom.

One day in the Oaxaca *alameda*, in the midst of sea of Christmas revelers, Marty and I came across a short, dark man from the Mixe, a cloud-shrouded, coffee growing highland. The man's pack contained strips of palm leaf, from which he rapidly fashioned a figure of an idealized raptor resembling a pteradactyl. I was enchanted with his creation. The price of one was ridiculously low, but believing that bargaining was obligatory in Mexico, I asked Marty to find out how much less he would charge if, let's say, I bought five. The man sullenly refused to hear of a discount. As I paused, confused about how to continue, the man began surveying the crowd for other customers. Martin then heatedly told me that this man probably made most of the cash he saw for the year by selling his creations to tourists for these few days. "The few cents you are trying to knock off each one is insignificant to you and very important to him. Either pay the price or let him get on to another customer." He was right. I felt ashamed as I watched the skill employed and the time it took to make the few I bought. I have the one he made for me to this day.

Gradually, we all incorporated the fact of Marty's chronic leukemia into our lives. Whatever flutter of fear was experienced when I thought of it was overpowered by the activity present at the time. Chronic lymphacytic leukemia became known as CLL to us all.

Until the winter of 1990/91. It was then that I first noticed that every time I talked to Marty on the telephone I would hear a blurry tone to his voice, muffled through a heavy cold. Most of his other signs were still in the range that he had lived with for almost two decades. He said he was feeling well. He said he was active and energetic. There were a few troubling differences between the past and now. His spleen, distended by the increasing quantity of immature white cells it could not adequately process, was larger than it had ever been -- you could see the bulge it made.

It became apparent over the next few months that something was wrong. The infection was diagnosed as recurrent sinusitis. Round after round of antibiotics did not seem to make a dent in it. Despite his assurances that he felt good, he sounded awful. Although he denied it at the time, he was fatigued much of the time. He'd get winded climbing up stairs. He had night sweats. His neutrophils (white blood cells that play a major role in the body's defense against bacteria, viruses and fungi) were dangerously low. Marty started pressing his doctor to find out what was going on and once again, after many years of silence on the subject, we started talking about a bone marrow transplant.

We were 56 years old. I was in good health, free from any diseases or conditions that would disqualify me as his bone marrow donor. Coloring that thought however, was that my health could change suddenly, or that I could die unexpectedly, leaving Marty without a donor. It seemed time to explore all possibilities. Could my marrow be extracted, frozen and stored until he needed it? Were we truly biologically identical? Marty contacted Dr. Joel Rappeport, a bone marrow transplant specialist he had consulted with some years prior and with whom he was very favorably impressed. He put his health care plan hematologist, his primary care physician and Dr. Rappeport in contact with each other.

His team was in place. They were talking to each other. New tests were ordered for Marty. He asked his health plan to consider him for a bone marrow transplant. I had blood drawn in Phoenix and sent to Boston to be tissue typed to make sure that we were still identical. We were.

For twenty years Marty lived with leukemia, which, although a dread disease, did very little to inhibit his activities or dampen his enjoyment of life. Now, in the parlance of the doctors, the biology of the disease had changed. What it meant to all of us, Marty's family, was that after being level all those years the trend for the future was downward, maybe precipitously so. The most dramatic symptom of the recent change was the sinus infection that plagued him. When they finally found an antibiotic that attacked the infection his symptoms would abate while he was taking the drug. The day after he stopped taking it his symptoms would reappear.

Arline and I traveled to Israel and Italy in September of 1991. On the return trip, with twenty or thirty minutes between planes in New York, I called Marty. I hadn't spoken to him in a little over three weeks. He was feeling well when we left. Nothing mystical about "having to call Marty," even at a moment when I was somewhat anxious about making our plane connection and fatigued from a long flight. No tingling feeling, no palpable prescience, no Corsican brothers reaction. I just felt strongly motivated to call him at that moment.

He told me that in the past week he had been in the M.I.T. infirmary undergoing treatment and tests because his neutrophil count had virtually gone to zero and he had developed a slight fever. He had been in great danger. His body had no power to resist infection. Had he not had medical attention immediately he could have been overwhelmed by infection and died. It was my first understanding of how shot his immune system was and how truly insidious his disease was. It also became plain that the bone marrow transplant was not a theoretical and distant possibility but something that more than probably would have to be done for Marty's survival.

Despite being weakened by the recurrent sinus infections and the unencouraging prognosis, Marty was living. He was teaching his courses as he had always done. He had just returned in early September from a four-country trip to Central America. Marty's interest in pure cultural anthropology had changed somewhat since the late seventies, diverging from the strictly academic to a more activist role. In time, building on his experience with Mexican peasants, he became an expert on agrarian reform, appearing before congressional committees and ultimately advising negotiators of the Salvadoran peace accords. He became an active advocate, attacking the Reagan policies toward Central America, writing editorials in newspapers across the country, appearing on radio and television and speaking on many campuses. His scholarly writing became limited to Central American matters.

His reputation spread. He was sought after to present the rebuttal to our government's policies in Central America, to give the leftist point of view. Widely traveled in the region, fluent in Spanish, well practiced in anthropological investigation, he was not a college freshman, newly liberated from his home, looking for a cause to make his blood boil. He was a seasoned social scientist, able with calm and articulate discussion, to make audiences understand what the real effects of our government's policies were on the lives of the *campesinos* of El Salvador, Nicaragua, Guatemala and Honduras. He made many trips to the area, meeting with people of every sector of society. He went to places accessible only by canoe or on foot as well as the air conditioned offices of high government officials. Everywhere he went he interviewed those he met, formally or informally.

His interest in the complex of problems in Central America, combined with his lifetime of formal study and field work, permitted him to synthesize his work into an activism supported by solid training. He excited his students, weaving current Latin American themes into the traditional fundamentals of anthropology. In the late eighties, the same edition of the M.I.T. newspaper that announced his elevation to full professor, described his arrest, along with some of his colleagues, in a demonstration against the Reagan policies.

As his health became more precarious his travel to Central America worried me. I thought, at the time, that Marty was denying his sickness too actively. I imagined his getting ill in rural Nicaragua or El Salvador and dying before he could receive even the most rudimentary treatment. In his case, it was possible. If he had contracted an infection just the month before when, as we now knew, he had virtually no neutrophils, he certainly would have died without sophisticated treatment. I couldn't help but think of Peter Davis. In his book *Where is Nicaragua?* He writes of being stricken with a bleeding ulcer while visiting in that impoverished, strife-ridden country. The medical advice he receives is to get back to the U. S. as fast as possible.

I was angry at Marty for not being more conservative with his health, for causing me to worry. But I knew in the same instant as I became angry with him that he could do nothing else but continue to live as he was used to and give us all assurances that he was stronger than he must have known, or at least felt, he was. Like the good social scientist he is, he went about investigating his own condition, methodically and honestly. His medical team was compiling the relevant information, analyzing it and drawing to a conclusion. In the meantime, he was not going to lie down and wait for an imagined end. He was not going to cooperate with the damned disease by behaving weakly. It was his way of fighting and while I was angry at him for making me worry, I loved him for it.

A therapeutic strategy was being developed; Marty would receive some rounds of chemotherapy. It would either be a curative or, more likely, a conditioner for the Bone MarrowTransplant. The number of treatments would be decided upon based on his reaction and tolerance to them. Before the transplant could take place however, his sinus infection had to be cleared up surgically. If the antibiotics could not defeat it, especially if it was fungal in origin, the medical reasoning went, and if it flared when Marty had lost his remaining defenses to the onslaught of the chemotherapy (and the radiation just before the transplant), he would have no resistance, no immune response and no white blood cells with which to marshall a defense.

Marty had the operation to clear out his sinuses, a kind of reaming out, a nasty piece of plumbing. A miniature roto-rooter was snaked inches up his nose and through his sinus passages and manipulated so that the blockage would be cut or ripped out. It left him raw and in pain for a much longer time than he was told to expect. To prevent hemorrhaging, his nose and sinuses were packed with a rubbery substance. That lasted some days, during which time he could not breathe through his nose at all. It meant that every time he fell asleep and his mouth closed involuntary, unable to draw air into his lungs, he would be startled awake.

He was in the hospital for several days and at home for weeks recovering. It was his first experience with surgery and the hospital. It depressed him

-- this look, this taste of the near future. It was probably also his first experience with feeling the effects in his own body of the euphemistic descriptions the doctors use to allay your fears. "Uncomfortable," "a few days of discomfort," "it will bother you some." It was much worse than that. They didn't tell about sleep deprivation, about the disorientation that inevitably comes in the transition from being healthy to being sick. I could hear the pain in his voice when he was able to talk to me, and what I thought at the time was his confusion at not being able to square his physical feelings with what they had told him to expect. If this rather simple, preparatory procedure like the sinus surgery caused as much pain and difficulty in recovery, what would the future hold for him. Could he tolerate it? Would he want to?

DECISIONS

During the flight to Boston to visit Marty I was made aware of the power of my gloom when I found I had been reading the same page for the longest time without comprehension. I closed the book, removed my glasses, let my shoulders sink back into the seat, shut my eyes and permitted the thoughts about Marty, held at bay by the book I was pretending to read, to come flooding into my mind. I hadn't seen him in almost a year. I pictured him frail, bald, fevered, sick. All from the chemotherapy he had just begun.

The image produced a tremor of fear in me that shattered the comfortably quiescent state into which I had settled. I was jarringly wide awake now, no longer interested in reading but not wanting to think the dark thoughts my mind fastened onto every time I thought of Marty. It was not difficult for me to both understand and feel the image of him failing. I didn't have to sift through my reading on the subject or to try to match what he was going through to some experience of mine. I knew.

The brilliantly white clouds flying slowly past the plane seemed so comforting, so soothing. Their fantastic, changing shapes distracted me momentarily, and I wished with a little boy's fervor that they would accompany me and defend me from the horror I believed was pursuing me: watching Marty in the grip of his wasting disease, being transformed into something that was not a part of me as death drew him further and further away, that I would stand, rooted in life, while he would fall.

The recent change in Martin's condition had come quickly. The many years of knowing about his leukemia and, at the same time, watching him live a relatively normal life led me to minimize the possibility that his disease would change as abruptly as it did. Over the years, as the fear of his dying diminished, it was gradually replaced by the comforting thought that he would live a normal span, that he would die of what would claim me, a disease that would be the consequence of old age. Now it was all changed. Because of the threat to Martin's life the thought of death was more understandable, more palpable, more proximate, more frightening.

The image of Martin dying did not form itself as a thought. It surged through my stomach. I became, for the instant, the little boy, crouched over; walking to school in the winter, trying to burrow deeper into his mackinaw to find the warmth that he believed would bring the relief from the pain in his stomach. The skinny, sallow stutterer, who could find succor neither at school nor at home with his parents.

Mr. Kirschbaum orders his fourth-grade class to settle down and writes the assignment on the blackboard. He sits at his desk and, for a moment or two, looks out over the classroom to make sure the children are at work on the task. He puts both of his feet on the top of his desk and opens the newspaper, obscuring his face. A tall man, slow of movement, his yellowish face never completely shaven, he moves grudgingly, without energy. He is one of a crop of young men whose careers had been interrupted by the war. His speech to the children is always sarcastic, tinged with violent forebodings.

After a few minutes the ugly game begins. Whispering erupts among the students, among the boys. Mr. Kirschbaum lowers the newspaper, exposing only his eyes. Thus, partially veiled, he surveys the now hushed room. "Let's see, who do I use for football practice today? You were talking, weren't you, Weiss?"

"No, it wasn't me," says the wiry Weiss, a theatrical, hurt look coming over his face.

"I'm never wrong twice in a row. Get up here, Diskin."

"Which one?" The class titters.

"You, which one are you?", he says, pointing at me, his black, dull, menacing eyes sighting down his finger.

"S-S-Saul."

"Get under my desk, S-S-Saul, and think about how to correct your behavior. A few minutes under there will clarify your thoughts."

A certain thrill goes through me as I assume the position under his small, Department of Education, standard issue desk. I am the outlaw, admired and pitied by my fellows. I had been there before, crouching in a corner of the wooden cell, making my body as small as possible, hoping to confuse him as to my precise position. I watch as Mr. Kirschbaum lowers his feet from the top of the desk and places them, deliberately, under the desk. I have a whiff of an

53

acrid, unclean odor. He continues reading the newspaper, now spread flat on the desk, slowly turning pages.

Sighing exaggeratedly and stretching his arms, his fists rising toward the ceiling, he kicks swiftly, without warning. He misjudges my position and his foot hits the modesty panel, making a loud, hollow, sound. The class laughs. Mr. Kirschbaum silences them with a venomous look. I had won the opening skirmish. I know he is angered by my trick and I fear what will follow. With his right leg he presses me into the left side of the desk.

"Mr. Kirschbaum, c-c-can I c-c-come out now?" I try to scourge my words of the fear I was trembling with.

"Do you hear something? It sounds like the squeak of a mouse. I wonder…" With that he lashes out with his left foot, hitting me behind the ear, the tip of his shoe caroming into the wood. From the sound the whole class knows he had hit me hard. A gasp arises.

A great, malevolent smile breaks over Mr. Kirschbaum's face. He bends under the desk and grasps me by the shoulder, leading me to me feet. I hold my head where he had kicked me, struggling not to cry.

"What on earth were you doing under my desk? Don't you know you can have an accident there?'

I go silently back to my seat and stare straight ahead, not wanting any acknowledgment of my humiliation. Tears leak down my cheek and I wish Mr. Kirschbaum dead. I know I can't seek the protection of my parents. If I tell them they will assume I did something to deserve the punishment. I don't want the pity of the girls in the class. I don't want the bravado commiseration of the boys. Everyone has seen me cry and heard me stutter. Only Marty knows how I feel. I don't have to tell him. His face is twisted into a grimace of tormented sympathy for me. He wants to avenge me, to strike out at Mr. Kirxchbaum but he cannot. He suffers as much as I do, even more.

My visit was a couple of months after the sinus surgery and about a week or so after the administration of the first dose of chemotherapy. It was May, 1992. I was anxious to find out if the chemotherapy had left any ravage on Marty's body. One of the side effects was that he was supposed to lose his hair. When we discussed it I could tell that it held a terror for Marty. If he became bald, even temporarily, it might make him feel sick and old and weak. In one of our phone conversations he told me, cheerily, that if went bald he would at last be able to use the vast collection of hats he had acquired over the years in various parts of the world. We clowned crazily together over the various disguises he would be able to assume.

I heard the landing gear grinding and the muffled voice of a flight attendant. Out of the window I saw the landing field at Logan Field, a finger of land protruding into the water, daring the Atlantic, and I thought of Marty with a shiver of fearful anticipation.

People coming to greet arriving passengers were required to wait behind a barrier at the end of the long, wide indoor avenue flanked by the waiting areas beyond which planes nose up to the terminal to receive and disgorge passengers. I would use the time required to walk the hundred yards or so before greeting Marty to settle myself. I found that I was almost twitching as if composing myself through my skin. I wanted to see Marty first, before he saw me. He had lost weight since I last had seen him - he was a little over 150 pounds compared to my 175 pounds. I didn't want to show surprise at his appearance. I strained to catch a glimpse of him to shrug off any look of shock I might have.

A hundred or so people were waiting. It was the usual Boston crowd; the North End young bloods and Southies in tee shirts, displaying bronzed, tattooed biceps, accompanied by their Angies and Teresas with extravagantly lustrous black or red hair and too tight dresses or jeans, university students dressed in Patagonia or Eddie Bauer, temperature-appropriate for the mid-May weather, blacks from the neighborhoods dressed in leather or fancy jogging outfits, an assortment of Asians and Hispanics, melded with the undistinguished, the people who could have been from any city, from any region, the generic. I peered intently into the crowd, between briefcases and backpacks, over heads, around hips. I heard Portuguese, I jerked my head in the direction of the Caribbean Spanish with swallowed consonants, expecting to see Marty with a puckish leer, saying something filthy to me in a Spanish he was sure I would not be able to understand. No Marty.

Where the fuck was he? I travel three thousand miles and I arrive on time and he can't time his goddamned thirty-minute trip to get here on time. I soften immediately, almost smiling.

Was he too sick to come, I thought with a stab? Did he become ill between the time I left Phoenix and the time I arrived in Boston? Or, was he just waiting below at the baggage carousel. I walked past the crowd after making two sallies through it and down the escalator to the baggage area. Still no Marty.

I decided to go back upstairs on the chance that he had simply arrived late yet gone to the appointed place. As I mounted to the upstairs level I could see him, agitatedly scanning the direction from where I had disembarked. I sidled up to him and from six inches away I patted his leather jacket and said, "Hi, Marty".

His worried look melted into a beaming smile. We hugged and kissed each other. I could feel how skinny he had become. The difference between 175 pounds and 150 pounds was meaningless until I felt how fragile and weak he appeared. I softened the pressure of the embrace I held him in for fear of hurting him, of breaking him.

Along the way to the parking garage Marty told me, with the slightly embarrassed way he has when he is feeling mildly guilty, that the traffic was heavy, that he misread the time and other such palpably transparent excuses. He was smiling as he was talking and so was I. We were both exulting in seeing each other again, in confirming that we were still both alive, that we were both together. In the elevator going up to the proper level in the parking garage, my eyes met his fully and glazed with tears. I reached over, drew his skinny face toward me, my hand gently brushing the bulging lymph node in his throat, and kissed his cheek. He was moved, and in a quavering voice he said,"Vane, vane" (Cry, Cry) one the Yiddish phrases we used when the English could not give the precise flavor of our thought. We were both slightly embarrassed, slightly uncomfortable. We were willing to be embarrassed or uncomfortable. We were not used to expressing ourselves to each other without reserve, without defenses. When we were children we didn't have to express ourselves openly. We knew precisely what the other was experiencing without words. After all the years of living apart, of living different lives, there was doubt about the other. We would have to be clear and open with each other. As the emotion subsided and the tears evaporated, and relieved that no one had surprised us crying and embracing on that grimy industrial elevator in the airport parking garage, I knew that that was what I wanted to recapture and what we both needed if I was to be of help to Marty. We would have to regain something of what we had as children, of being twins again. As children it served us well to prepare for the world we would face. Now it could help us stave off death.

Memory is a river. In its youth it courses wildly, propelled by vigor, eager for the future, shouting greetings at the mountain sky. It travels varied and unexpected terrain toward its final amalgamation with the ocean, with a delta, a formless swamp or savannah, with death. Along the way it changes. It joins other streams. It dives faster, it flattens and slows, it becomes muddy and then clear again. And it always changes, is changed, by its surroundings. Its water becomes alkaline, then acid, now rich with suspended nutrients, generously supporting teeming life, now becoming sterile and impoverished, host only to tenacious, deformed survivors. It alternately hides and reveals itself. It dies and is born again, sometimes refreshed and revitalized, but more often chastened, repentant, saddened, exhausted.

Just as the river water changes in its journey, so do the experiences of life change the recollection of past events. Memory is not camera-like objective or irrefutably certain. It cannot be. Too much is at stake for it to be. Between people whose lives are intertwined, who have shared intense experience or been present at the same events in the past, memory differs, particularly over matters of great emotional importance. Not simply in a self-serving way but in a way that means that the perception of those events, the experience of them was, and remains, different.

Someone said that memory is hidden treasure. Sometimes, perhaps. Sometimes it is a wound unhealed, not often thought of, not brought to the fore of consciousness, just left to lie dormant with the hope that it will never again rise to give pain. Memories of triumphant feats, of successes, become aggrandized, amplified, delicious to recall, sweetening the present. Those moments will exist forever, growing in appreciation with recall.

Defeats, humiliations, failures, lapses of character, can also never be erased, just suppressed, distorted and forgotten. They surface in memory as regret, corrosive, shameful reminders that can only poison the present.

Between Marty and me it is even more complicated. Of certain events we share memories that are all but identical. Of certain episodes, certain happenings, certain moments we remember every detail, every nuance, every descriptive particular, except one central fact—which one of us experienced it. Marty will swear it happened to him and I will do the same. We both mean it. We are both right. If an event was so important that it lingered in memory and was retold from time to time, then it does not matter who experienced it and who observed it. We were equally effected by it and, in the most real sense, it happened to both of us.

Our conversation began as soon as the car cleared the parking garage. We proceeded immediately in a straightforward, business-like manner. Information, hard, distressing facts needed to be conveyed, and soon. If we waited until we got home there would be more greetings, embraces, welcomes, that in turn would lead to questions about our families, nostalgic remembrances. By that time food and drink would dominate the rest of the evening. I was only going to be there for a couple of days. Marty had told me that we were all invited to a dinner party. The evening would be so normal, so full of the warmth of seeing each other again, of laughter, that discussion of disease and of its long term consequences would be something easy to put off.

"How are you feeling?"

The joy of greeting and the emotional comfort given by seeing each other retreated in the face of the question. Marty's thumb jerked on the steering wheel, the residue of a persistent childhood tic. "Pretty good. I get tired quickly. I'm glad the semester is over."

"Any side effect from the chemotherapy?" I was afraid to include the word "yet" in the question.

"Nothing yet. I'm sure it's just too early to tell. The first one was just a few days ago." As you can hear, my nose crap is not entirely cleared up even after that damn nose reaming. Every few days I start hawking stuff out of my nose that I can barely believe when I look at my tissue. It looks like mice and twigs and boulders. When I'm done it feels like I've cleaned out the sinuses forever. In a few days it's back. You know, on the one hand I'm glad that the chemotherapy hasn't made my hair fall out or made me sick to my stomach but it's my understanding that if it doesn't do those things it's not producing results. "A friend of ours in Phoenix called me a few months ago to tell me she was sorry that you were sick. I quickly told her that you weren't sick, that the biology of your disease had changed, that you were undergoing a series of evaluations to see what the new therapeutic strategy should be and that you're trying to determine whether a bone marrow transplant is necessary."

He gave me a look intended to convey blunt truth before he answered. "She was right. I am sick. I can't concentrate. If I start reading something, I fall asleep in minutes. I drag myself around. I haven't done any work on my book in the longest time. I've got to have the transplant, man." He said it deliberately, an assertion not to be questioned.

We cleared the multi-laned exit road and moved swiftly along the boulevard leading out of the airport and abruptly entered the cruelty of Boston traffic. Marty concentrated on the driving, letting me know by his manner that I was not required to comment on what he had just told me. I didn't want to answer or comment. I just wanted to think and absorb. We crawled in the lava-flow approach to the Callahan tunnel till it narrowed into two lanes in the tunnel itself. The familiar sound of the horns blaring in the tunnel, usually irritating, was pleasantly distracting, almost friendly.

As soon as we emerged into the soft, faded, afternoon light leading toward the broad reach of the upward sloping entrance to the expressway a long line of cars slowed us to an annoying crawl. It was obvious that there was some obstruction. Fifteen or twenty cars ahead we could see two cars immobilized. As we drew near we could see that both were taxi cabs. The drivers were standing near their respective cabs, each guarding his territory, arguing. The car in front was commanded by a beefy, red-faced man with a large, protruding belly, a veteran Boston cabby. He stood toward the back of his car facing the much younger black driver who had one leg inside his cab, the other on the road. His accent was Jamaican.

"Dere ain't no damage, mon. Why don' you just drive away and stop holding up traffic?"

"You just get off the fuckin' boat, someone hands you a license and you're tellin' me what to do. A shit-for-brains jerkoff like you, tellin' me what to do. When the cops get here they'll tell you what to do."

The front bumper of the black man's cab was a couple of inches from the rear bumper of the other cab. There did not appear to be any damage to either car. Both men were sweating.

"Please, mon, dis costing us both money just standing here."

"You'll find out about costing money," he replied oblivious to the traffic jam being caused, a smile beginning.

We finally made it around the cars obstructing traffic and mounted the entrance to the expressway. I could see the Charles River and the buildings of Harvard and M.I.T. The scattered clouds in the late afternoon western sky were backlit a bright silver by the descending sun. A pure and comforting light, it contrasted with the foul, noisy traffic, with its insistent smell and confusion, and it made the immediate, the near, the buildings, the cars and the river seem unclean and disheveled, while the far pristine, clean and full of hope.

My mind was crowded with pictures of the future, most of them dire and miserable. Words and scenes and acts flooded my mind; speeches, cries of lamentation, orations of defiance and anger. I wanted desperately to say something wise, soothing, something healing and clever at the same time.

"What did you think about the riots in Los Angeles?"

"You mean the uprising?"

We both smiled, neither one of us looking at the other. We rode in silence, smiling. There would be time to take up the challenge, the contest in which politics was the metaphor. It would get heated later in the visit. It always did. For now, a tiny jab, a needle, easily deflected, with no harm done. No winner, no loser. Maybe, because of the special circumstances of this visit and its brevity, we would get through it with no strong argument.

Marty and Vilunya, (who changed her name from Wilma some years before), live in Lexington, Massachusetts, 30 minutes from Boston, when traffic cooperates. Their house, built around 1740, looks like the rural manor house it was when it was attached to the farming acreage surrounding it. Today it is surrounded by homes of a more recent vintage, "ranches," "Cape Cods," "Victorians," both real and copied. Theirs is the last house on a street that terminates in a cul-de-sac. Just beyond, hidden from view by dense greenery, is an expressway. Looking through an upstairs window at the vegetable garden or the hillside of original forest interspersed with newly planted trees, both decorative and fruit bearing, one can see the 18th century while the ear confirms the end of the 20th.

I always like coming to their house, especially at this time of the year. The earliest possible time to plant a vegetable garden, May 30th, was still two weeks away. Time enough for a late frost. The air was fresh and crisp, a little chilly for me in the evening and early morning. The natural surroundings had an explosive fecundity, an achingly green smell everywhere. Looking from the lawn to the wild hillside every shrub and tree seemed poised for the new cycle. Some of the buds on the trees and bushes were swollen, presaging the momentary offering of sweet odor and brilliant color. The earth of the vegetable garden was tilled and ready to receive seeds and seedlings, its dark brown ground looking and smelling healthy.

Vilunya came to greet us as we entered the enclosed porch leading to the front door. She was smiling with her whole face, her eyes glowing with greeting as we hugged and kissed. We held hands and looked at each other for a few seconds and hugged again. Marty stood to the side and beamed.

"I'm so glad to see you. It's been a long time".

"Yes, it's great to be here." I felt slightly ill at ease, trembly. I didn't know why. Perhaps fatigue from the long trip. Perhaps anticipating being immersed in a subject I wished I didn't have to deal with.

She took my arm and drew me to her. "Come in, come in, let's not stand in the doorway all day. Sit down, you look a little tired. Can I get you something? Hungry?"

"Actually, what I'd love is a drink. Let me just put my bag away and take off my jacket. Am I upstairs near Aaron's room?"

The Bloody Mary I'd had on the plane left me with an oily taste in my mouth. What I wanted was something that would relax my brain and tame the devils I had been conjuring. I carried my bag upstairs, surveyed the room and sat on the bed to collect myself. I opened the window slightly to let some air circulate and sat on the bed again. The room felt stuffy. I let myself sag, sink on the bed, with drooping shoulders, my unease being replaced by a light feeling, akin to optimism. My sight and touch had confirmed that Marty was alive. I washed my hands and face on the way downstairs.

The house itself looked close to its original shape, I am told, even after two and a half centuries and despite numerous remodeling, additions and modernizations. There were still places where original clinch nails could be found. With the exception of the construction they had done since they bought the house there did not seem to be a single wall that was plumb nor a single floor that was level. The first few times I was in the house I felt slightly disoriented, almost having a touch of vertigo. It felt as if I might fall off the floor.

I joined Marty and Vilunya in the expansive kitchen and dining room. Remodeled several years before, it was a graceful room, skillfully finished, bright and airy. I felt a renewal of energy. Rubbing my hands together theatrically I asked where the booze was.

"Rum okay, Sauly? I've got a great Haitian rum." Marty poured the rum into a couple of glasses and we both sampled our drink. Sighing appreciatively, we sat at the dining table.

"A lot has happened since you were here last, Saul," said Vilunya with an expression that changed from gayety to seriousness.

"Yeah. Marty's been telling me a little about it driving here and I know the headlines from phone conversations. I'm anxious to know all the details. How are you feeling about it all?"

Vilunya's face grew taut. She looked directly in front of her at the table. Her voice lowered. Her tone flattened. I was not looking at Marty but I could feel his concentration on Vilunya's words.

"All right so far. Naturally, it scares me, thinking about it, not knowing precisely how it will unfold. We're gathering information, trying to learn as much about it as possible." Her voice trailed off and she looked past me, out of the window, as if she were trying to recapture a thought that had eluded her for the moment, a thought pleasanter than the one at hand.

Vilunya was orphaned in the Second World War. She was the only one of her family from Poland who survived the Nazi slaughter. When she was about two years old a servant of her family took her into her household to raise along with her own children so she could not be distinguished as a Jewish child. She was uprooted from that family after the war and given to a rabbi and his wife. They wandered about, spending some time in a displaced persons camp, always living in cramped and squalid quarters. Finally, in 1948, they were able to cross to the U.S., where she was adopted by a well-to-do family. She had been given the name Wilma when she was brought to the U.S. as being a close approximation of her eastern European name. As an adult she decided to change her name to acknowledge her background and chose Vilunya.

Losing everyone she depended on and loved early in life had left its mark on her. Now, the possibility of losing Marty, with whom she had lived almost her entire adult life, must have dredged up her darkest fears. As I looked at her the image formed in my mind of the little girl whose tiny hand, held above her head, is enfolded in the grasp of an adult. Her hand is too small to grasp the much larger one. She can only hope that the adult hand hers is in, will not let go, will not leave her again. She is dragged as baggage across a ravaged landscape, through shabby, makeshift government offices, sleeping in cold and dangerous places, waiting in barren and desolate sites of temporary refuge, waiting, always waiting for her case to be resolved, for the grown-ups to let her stay in one place, to rest, to play, to be taken care of, to be loved. She brought her gaze back to the table, her focus returning.

"From everything I've heard the chances of success are great. We just have to make sure the transplant is absolutely necessary. It still involves a lot of risk."

I flashed a look at Marty. He met my look with one that told me that, although he was sure the transplant was necessary, Vilunya was not quite ready to acknowledge it to herself. I would know how to behave.

The dinner was at Susanna's house in Cambridge. She was a colleague of Marty's, a professor of anthropology and friend of many years. She was well known for her cooking; elaborate, traditional dishes not usually encountered outside of expensive restaurants. I had been at other dinners she had given that coincided with my visits and I was pleasantly anticipating the meal that awaited. Many years before, when my experience of food was still limited to basic fare, I was served a Provencal garlic soup at Susanna's.

She lived in a cramped apartment at the time and people were balancing plates and bowls on laps and knees. The broth of the garlic soup was exquisite. At the bottom of the bowl was something that felt to my spoon like a lump of bread, which, if true, would be infused with the lovely garlic flavor I was regretting coming to an end of. I scooped the whole clot up in the spoon and placed it in my mouth and chewed several times before I ascertained that it was pure garlic, cooked somewhat, to be sure, but nevertheless, a golf ball of garlic. It had not lost much of its power in the cooking. I could feel the heat begin to spread in my mouth as I chewed it hastily and swallowed it. My entire head started to heat up. I was sure everyone there could see the bright red color my face was turning. I thought I was going to faint. I was incapable of speech. No one else in the room had a similar reaction and it mortified me to know that I was the only one not sophisticated enough to know that the lump of garlic was to be left in the bottom of the bowl, not eaten.

I was glad to be going to Susanna's house. It would be a festive interlude in the next days largely devoted to talking about Marty's health. In addition to looking forward to the meal I was interested in seeing the interaction between Marty and his friends. How would they react to the deterioration of his health? Did they know? Were they close enough so that they would be expected to know? Certainly Nate, an English professor and Marty's close friend, would know.

Marty and Vilunya told me that Nate and Susanna had recently taken up together. It seemed an improbable combination to me. Susanna, thin, good looking and well groomed, was spare in her speech and highly disciplined. She seemed slightly shy, withdrawn. She listened more than she spoke. To her it was a question of manners that you did not compete, with rising voice, to speak. She appeared to be the model of decorum. Nate had a loud opinion about everything. He was confident and loose, his posture a slouch, his language a weapon. He would eye the other participants in a discussion, surveying them for weakness while waiting his turn. Sometimes, before his turn, his voice would slash through the speaker's with a devastating point. He was smart and tough in argument and I could feel the tension build in the room when he became engaged. Marty told me that Nate was cosmopolitan, European. He could make himself comfortable wherever he went. He knew wine, good food, the most scenic routes, the best places to vacation. He was the child of Jewish refugees who fled the Nazis. I smiled at the thought of the combination.

I looked forward to the evening for another reason. In past years occasions like this would sometimes leave me burning. I would have come from Phoenix, where politics was not followed and discussed obsessively as it was in Cambridge. Even in ultra-conservative Arizona the left, from liberal to radical, was not derided with the seeming hatred I heard Marty's friends refer to the right. While my political opinions were generally similar to theirs, the vehemence with which they expressed them always made me feel attacked, uncomfortable. In my daily life I was surrounded by people whose views were conservative, who were almost always on the opposite side of political issues from me. They were not fascists or bloodsuckers. They were people like me, struggling, trying to make a living, full of doubts about the world and one's chances for succeeding in it.

In those days, the sixties, the academics who railed against the right lived better than I did at the time, much better. They earned considerably more than I did at well paying jobs with rich benefits. Money for extras such as travel abounded, money for anything which could be characterized as research despite the lax standards applied for evaluation. Everyone, it seemed had entertaining stories to tell of frauds on the university, on the government. Only they were never characterized as frauds, merely as amusing vignettes, such as the doctoral candidate investigating the Sikhs of Fresno, California, pocketing the portion of his grant for housing and sleeping in his car. No one was hurt. Just the ugly, unworthy, *them*, the bureaucrats, the institutions of oppression, the unfeeling defenders of the corrupt establishment. Those were good times for academics but it didn't seem to me that they had much charity for the rest of us.

That was in the sixties and early seventies. I was finding it hard to make a living in the real estate business, my trade. In one of my visits I heard a discussion about whether apartment rents in Cambridge should be controlled by law. There were mass meetings, raging public debates, appearances at the Cambridge city council, a newsletter in which one of the large apartment owners was constantly referred to as Superpig Wasserman. I wondered how the users of that phrase could have expected to negotiate seriously with someone they had just insulted. I felt closer to Wasserman than I did to Marty's friends.

I also marveled at how little they seemed to know about the life of ordinary people; about what they did for a living, where they lived. A familiar exchange at the time when I was introduced for the first time to a friend of Marty's was,

"Where do you teach?"

"I don't teach. I'm a businessman."

"What kind of business?"

"Real estate."

"Where do you live?"

"Phoenix, Arizona."

"How interesting."

Exotic to a provincial Easterner perhaps. Out of the realm of their experience perhaps, but by every signal given off by the questioner, by the lack of any follow-up question or discussion, certainly not interesting. Sometimes to be polite, I felt, people would ask questions about Arizona. Those questions almost always betrayed a profound ignorance of the place except to regard it only as the nether reach of Goldwater country. Some of these were people who were well aquainted with regions and cities across the world. Those were interesting places. Arizona was not. Nebraska, Ohio were not. In the many years that have since passed I have become less prickly on the subject and have lost the envy for their lives I once had. I have seen many of them tempered by raising and educating children, straining to pay a mortgage and, after the excitement that their work used to give them diminished to the habitual, struggle to discover other interests that could fulfill them. Just like the rest of us.

Susanna's dinner party was civilized, pleasant and relaxing, terms that would not have been complimentary many years ago. The ten people or so were all academics or married to one, with the exception of me. There were no wildly invigorated conversations, no strong arguments. The guests that I had never met before were more than polite to me. I sensed that they knew about Marty's current state of health and as his twin brother they accorded me an extra ration of camaraderie and respect. Everyone knew, not only where Arizona was, but a great deal about its geography, its Indian reservations, it's current bizarre politics. I felt pleased about that. Not entirely in a chauvinistic way. Just the slightest bit smug that the place where I had lived for the past thirty years was being discovered.

Marty's illness was not discussed much. There were a few questions about his present state, mostly from Nate who wanted to know the precise effects of the chemotherapy so far. Some of the others present simply inquired about how he was, one with rather grave inflection to the words.

The evening's conversation followed the familiar pattern of the middle class, I thought with some irony. Most of the talk centered on the food and drink. How to cut and serve Susanna's lovely *Salmon en croute*, how long to breathe a wine, whether the Burgundy we were drinking, called simply

Bourgogne Rouge was a much better wine than the label indicated. A fair amount of time was devoted to discussing academic affairs, politics, and related gossip. And children, yes children, a subject seemingly banished from discussion years before, at least in my memory. Most of the people in the room had children in college or about to enter college or just finishing college and facing the outside world for the first time. The social uncertainties and the diminishing economic opportunities that our children faced were of great concern to all of us.

The pre-dinner talk hummed away in a comfortable living room that communicated through bay windows to the tree-lined street below. As the light faded from the outside and was replaced by lamplight inside, everyone achieved the first level of comfort bestowed by the knowledge that the company was comfortable and harmonious and the alcohol was producing the first, soft, feeling of relaxation.

The only political topic was Central America. Although it had faded considerably from the public interest since the election of 1990 that removed the Sandinistas from power, the subject had great currency in that room. Marty held everyone's attention.

Analysis. That was the most prized of all. Because most in the room were social scientists, hard data was both difficult to come by and agree upon. To arrive at the truth one had to do more than compile or present fact. The data had to be interpreted, to be analyzed subtly, skillfully, so that the conclusion would be persuasive and seemingly consensual. Marty was a master at it. He did it quietly, with absolute authority, presaging in his listener's mind that behind every comment, every speculation, every conclusion, was a complex and well thought out argument supported by a mountain of proof. I listened with admiration to his description of the current conditions in Central America. Everyone in the room agreed with Marty.

Because everyone there was highly trained and educated the discussion at times sounded beautiful to me. It gave me a mild regret at not having it available to me for most of my adult life. And then I thought with a surge of inner mirth that exactly that same elegance of expression and complexity of analysis had been used many times by the same people, with the same serious earnestness, to analyze the basketball playoffs and the September Red Sox let down.

As the evening ended, all the guests bunched near the door to say good-byes. Two by two, handshakes and embraces punctuated the leavetaking. Susanna and Nate received the parting comments and told everyone how welcome they were. We were the last to leave. Nate kissed Marty on the lips.

"That's how we say goodbye to each other," he said, looking at me.

Marty appeared the slightest bit ill at ease. Nate was still focusing on me, as if I was supposed to express some opinion about his gesture. Something coarse and sarcastic flew into my mind but I said nothing.

The loose plan for the next morning was to have a large waffle breakfast and if the weather was good, to walk through a nature conservation area nearby. Marty was not awake when I came downstairs in the morning. The kitchen was swathed in the rich odor of coffee. Vilunya greeted me and offered me coffee. I poured it myself and sat at the table across the large kitchen.

"I'll be with you in a couple of minutes," she said. She was energetically preparing for breakfast: cutting oranges, arranging bowls and mixer for the making of the batter, which was to be ceremoniously performed by Marty.

I studied her while she worked. Of medium height and weight, her movements were quick and graceful. She attended to the task at hand with dedication. Her face was flat, with round cheeks and small nose, the face of an Asian nomad. Her dark brown hair, always dancing with light, framed her face perfectly. When she worked her concentration showed in a slight pinching up of her face. Even when she said she was listening to you while she worked it was obvious that her mind was only on her work. She expressed everything in her face. When a disappointment was felt her face fell, her eyes clouded with dismay. When something pleasant was happening such as a new person to meet, a trip to plan, her teeth all shown; her cheeks became two levitating, ripe apples and her eyes glowed with delight.

Especially when she was talking about her beloved Latin American folk art She knew a great deal about both the traditional and modern, particularly fabrics, which she talked about with a sensuous glow. In fulfillment of a long held goal she had opened a gallery and shop, which became well known in the Boston area and beyond.

Her love of Latin American folk art began during the three years of field work Marty did in southern Mexico. There Vilunya first encountered the culture that captivated her. She learned Spanish. She learned the ways of Mexican culture and society. Confident and unafraid, she would go to the native markets in the Guatemala highlands to buy goods for her shop. She loved it.

Marty entered the kitchen in his best bathrobe over pajamas and wearing lambhide slippers. He was shaved and showered, his black hair glistening.

"*Guten morgen*, Reb Tsalal," he said, extending his hand in my direction.

"*A shaine tog*, Reb Moshe," I said. We both bowed and grasped the tips of the fingers on the other's hand.

Marty was playing our father, dead eight years now. As children we delighted in Dad's Sunday morning ritual. It was the only day of the week he didn't work. He arose late and performed his bathroom ablutions leisurely. The steam from his hot shower seeped under the bathroom door to the adjoining room in our tiny apartment in Brooklyn. We could hear him singing Russian songs as he washed and shaved. When, at last, he left the bathroom in his bathrobe, headed for the kitchen and breakfast, a cloud, redolent of soap and shaving cream, filled the apartment. He was always in an uncharacteristically good mood, relaxed by the steam and self pampering. He kidded with Marty and me, tickling us while we struggled to escape. He made what we later thought to be lewd jokes with our mother in Russian. She would blush and after a time would say to him, "Oh, Moish." On Sunday morning the radio in the cramped kitchen was always tuned either to a Yiddish or Russian language program. When a favorite Russian song was being played he would sometimes join in, conducting the music with his fork, and when the feeling surged in him, he would leap to his feet and dance wildly to a Russian folk tune, his feet flying in an intricate step, one hand behind his neck, the other in the air, his eyes skyward, remembering a vodka-driven dance of horsemen around a fire, a rare, happy moment of his youth.

Marty fell to work on the waffle batter, explaining, in comic lecture for my benefit, the importance of every step in its preparation. He did it quickly, with practiced surety. When he was finished he sat down at the table with a cup of coffee and said that the batter had to rest a while before it would be ready to be transformed into perfect waffles.

"Is now a good time to talk about you, about the transplant? If it isn't let's figure out a good time. I'm nervous as hell about the subject but I'll feel even worse if I leave without having spoken about it with you."

Marty lowered and cocked his head slightly as if he were going to pull the answer out of some depth. I hadn't intended to change the mood quite so abruptly but I couldn't think of any more delicate way to do it. I realized, as I was waiting for his answer, that my heart was pounding fiercely. The air in the room became thin. Vilunya stared at her coffee cup and with her index finger ritually traced the rim of her cup over and over again.

Marty snugged his bathrobe around him. "I suppose now is as good a time as any. Let's talk at least till the batter is ready. The story is this; since I began feeling badly early last year we've been talking to the doctors about therapeutic strategies. I finally got my lead doctor in the health plan, Dr. Wellington, to start talking and corresponding with Joel Rappeport at the Yale-New Haven Center. You'll remember that I had contacted Rappeport in 1986, I think, as a result of a recommendation from my hematologist at the time. He came over to the house one Saturday and talked to Vilunya and me. He spent a couple of hours and, at the time, he sounded pretty certain that I was not ready for a transplant. We were both impressed, not only with his reputation and knowledge of the subject, but with his humanity. He was a real *mensch.*

"Beginning last fall, at about the time I was hospitalized with an infection and no neutrophils, I had to face the fact that I was getting sicker and sicker. Night sweats, fatigue, these constant respiratory infections. My health plan doctor and Rappeport began to believe that the disease was changing and that it was time to start talking seriously about a transplant. That's when I asked you to do those blood tests in Phoenix and we confirmed that our tissue types are identical."

I realized as he was talking that Marty and I had gone over this ground many times over the phone and that I was hearing everything he was saying as filler, as a preamble to the one question I wanted answered unequivocally; was the transplant on, and if so, when would it happen. I must have been fidgeting in my seat or my face must have shown something that Marty understood instantly.

"Look, everything the doctors say to me is conditional. This depends on that and that depends on this. Since last fall and winter, in fact since I got back from Central America early last September, all the docs have been talking about the transplant as if it should happen if we can work out the details. Where will it happen? What therapies should be used to prepare for it? Will the health plan pay for it? If so, what are their requirements? Is there a great rush to do it since I've got the best possible donor standing by? What happens if my donor suddenly gets hit by a bus? Should we look into cryonics for your marrow? Vilunya and I have looked at a couple of transplant facilities in Boston and we're going to New Haven to see Rappeport's facility."

Marty stopped speaking and took the last sip of his cold coffee and looked directly at me. "Everything I've just told you notwithstanding, and all the talk we've had over the last year about the science of my case doesn't make me capable of giving you a diagnosis or a prognosis. I may sound fluent in this subject but that's because I'm struggling to stay in the conversation with the doctors. All I can tell you, Sauly, is that I'm getting sicker and weaker and I feel like I'm going to die unless I get the transplant." He looked exhausted by his words. I felt something begin to break inside of me, like a rotting piece of lumber weakening a structure. Vilunya made a gurgling sound and abruptly went to the sink and vigorously washed her cup.

Marty rose and went slowly across the room to the waffle batter. He didn't look fresh and bathed any longer. He looked tired. He surveyed us, Vilunya crying quietly at the sink and I, still sitting at the table struggling with my composure and said with a crooked faced grin, "Let's have some waffles."

I'm the older of the two of us. By half an hour. It never meant much to either one of us except when we kidded about who got the birthright as in the biblical story read to us as children by our father. I would puff myself up and tell him I demanded respect because I was the older. He would say that he booted me out of the womb so he didn't have to share the warm spot. It was a routine we did for others usually, for people who asked us which one was older. There was always an edge to it, though, a not quite serious, not exactly unfunny air to it, a small relief when it was over. Marty and I never talked about it, never explored its meaning. I felt its meaning now. I was glad to be the oldest now. I was glad that I was the one he could depend on, that I could help him live. Marty had asked me sometime in the past year, in a phone conversation, if I would be his donor if he needed the transplant. He asked me formally, to get it out of the way. I told him I would. He thanked me. It was done rather briskly. I barely remember the conversation. He had to ask for the sake of planning. I had to answer. Between Marty and me it was a minor piece of business.

We all recovered during breakfast. I squeezed oranges, Vilunya made toast, heated syrup, brought the jams and cheeses to the table and Marty cooked the waffles. The political discussion started during the preparation and continued during breakfast.

We discussed as we ate. We made points as we passed the syrup or the yogurt. We rebutted the other with mouths full of waffles. Our mood improved. It was what we needed. Washing the meal down with the last of the strong coffee we all felt better, if slightly distended. We covered the presidential campaign. Marty, while supporting Clinton, and liking some of his ideas, found him too conservative. Vilunya was more enthusiastic about Clinton; she declared that he had genuine respect for women. Making some inward, obscene conclusions about his respect for women I allowed that I would hold my nose and vote for him. We covered other current subjects; the breakup of Yugoslavia, the Israeli-Palestinian peace discussions, the downsizing of American business, the globalization of labor. We agreed about none of them, although there was a twinkling acknowledgment between us that the argument offered by the other had some tiny validity, some minor point or two worth considering.

"What were the people in Watts rising against?"

Marty cocked his head in my direction before answering, smiling conspiratorially. "The proximate cause, the precipitant, as you well know, was the Rodney King verdict. The conditions that hadn't changed since the 70's'were the real underlying cause."

"An uprising sounds like the execution of a plan. Could you see any plan?"

"Not in the sense you mean. Maybe, more a way to shock whites. Remember what that guy who ran Operation Bootstrap in Watts said, 'we can have all kinds of self-help programs, neighborhood beautification, youth and job programs...nobody gives a damn. Let a black kid throw a rock through a window and Whitey takes notice.'"

"But what kind of notice? When the white majority sees looting, sees a white truck driver getting his brains beaten in by a black with a brick, how sympathetic do you think they're going to be?"

"Don't look for a well thought out plan with a clear agenda for social change to come from the people who are the victims of oppression."

"Victims of oppression? Of course there is injustice and prejudice, but you make South Central sound like Soweto, for god's sake."

"It's not far from it. Aside from the cultural differences, it's functionally not much different."

"Now I'm going to get a lecture in Anthropology?"

"What do you have to offer, a lesson on the virtues of laissez-faire capitalism?"

"No, what I have to offer you is a kick in the ass."

"Oh, yeah?"

71

"Yeah, and double yeah!"

Vilunya banged on a pot, a great smile on her face. "Boys, boys, you're wasting time. Let's go for a walk while the weather's good."

The rest of the visit, through the following day, was sweet and pleasant. We laughed and cackled and, in moments of lull, filled each other in on our respective lives. I left the next day with a gentle, pleasant ache, not with fear for the future or sorrow at Marty's condition or even the weight of what I now certainly knew to be my obligation. Just that it had been wonderful to see Marty and that I would miss him. A sweet, heavy, overflowing feeling. The perfect way to end a visit.

Leukemia is really quite simple to understand, unless, of course, it's your leukemia or the sufferer is one you love. Then it is too complicated to understand because you are convinced that there is a fact, a circumstance, a mitigant peculiar to your case that changes the grisly prognosis. And, unless you are a doctor yourself, the more you try to delve into the particulars of the subject, the more you try to understand the reasoning behind every diagnosis, every recommendation for therapy, the more confusing it becomes for you. In my case I obsessively tried to understand every step of the way. I read monographs on the subject, I asked endless questions of Marty and Vilunya and of various doctors, some attending Marty, others not. I became discouraged. I doubted my ability to understand what I was reading. I doubted my commitment to discovering the truth. Sometimes I asked the wrong questions. Sometimes I asked questions using the wrong terms, the wrong frame of reference. Sometimes I just didn't know what I was talking about. At times I asked questions to which there were no answers. Many of the questions I asked were in reality pleas for reassurance, for comfort, for Daddy to tell me all will be well.

A long way into the process I realized that I could never know enough about this constantly changing subject to satisfy myself and it calmed me somewhat. Instead I listened more to Marty, to the clinical information he gave me and, more importantly, to what he was experiencing. I had the broad outline understanding of the subject, enough to be able to follow along. He had plenty of doctors, most of whom he had confidence in. He needed an ally, not another medical voice. It was more important to defeat leukemia than to understand it.

Leukemias are cancers of the body's blood-forming tissues including the bone marrow and lymph system. These cancers cause the formation of large amounts of abnormal white blood cells, or leukocytes and are of two types; granulocytes (sometimes referred to as neutrophils), and lymphocytes. They both play a major role in the body's defenses against disease producing bacteria, viruses and fungi. The neutrophils rid the body of harmful bacteria and other foreign particles by engulfing and destroying them. The number of these white cells in the blood increase rapidly when needed to combat infection and usually return to normal once the infection is overcome.

Lymphocytes act in a different way. When the body is invaded by viruses or bacteria, the lymphocytes and other specialized cells respond by producing antibodies, substances that react with the invading infectious agent, or antigen, to ultimately destroy it and remove it from the body. Because each antibody is generally effective against only one type of antigen, different ones must be produced to combat each one. Memory cells are produced so that re-exposure to the same antigen provides a more rapid and efficient response.

Leukemia-caused abnormal white blood cells reach high concentrations in the bone marrow, lymph system, and blood stream, and their accumulation can interfere with the functions of vital organs. Eventually they overwhelm the production of healthy blood cells and platelets. Leukemia cell overproduction impairs the marrow, which is then unable to maintain production of sufficient numbers of red cells, platelets and healthy white cells. The net effect is anemia, bleeding and impaired infection-fighting capabilities. The deficiency in red blood cells means that the body's organs do not receive enough oxygen; the shortage of platelets makes the blood clotting process less effective, leaving the body more vulnerable to bleeding and bruising. As leukemic cells circulate through the body and lymphatic system, they infiltrate vital organs like the spleen and liver, which, in turn become impaired and cannot function properly. Often these organs become enlarged. Because of all of these effects, Leukemia is fatal without successful treatment.

There are acute forms of leukemias and chronic forms. The acute forms are intense, of fast onset and come to a crisis quickly. These leukemias affect immature cells still involved in the growth process. The chronic forms take longer to develop and are lingering. Chronic lymphocytic leukemia (CLL) refers to a malfunction in the production of lymphocytes which have reached a relatively mature stage of development.

CLL leads to the failure of the immune system. As the disease progresses the enfeebled immune system is no longer able to prevent the body from being overwhelmed by infection. CLL is understood to be moving rapidly when there are great increases in lymphocytes in the blood and marrow, enlarged lymph nodes, enlarged spleen and/or liver, anemia and low platelet count. Infections, even minor ones, require immediate treatment. Platelet transfusions are sometimes required to control bleeding problems.

Marty's counts were all going to hell. His white count was too high, all the others too low. CLL had sneaked up on him over this past year after quietly lying in wait for almost twenty years. It was now more powerful than the rest of this man called Marty. It would have to be killed soon or there would be no Marty.

The first of many vigils began. Chemotherapy was the first step in the plan that would probably lead to the bone marrow transplant. "Would probably" instead of certainly, because now Marty was entering uncharted territory and it was impossible to predict how his body would react. One of the possibilities, remote to be sure, was that the chemotherapy he had started would lead to a remission that would last the rest of his life, or at least that was a hope harbored by some of us. His disease had been controlled for almost twenty years with the drugs chlorambucil and prednisone. The chemotherapy he had just started was known by the acronym, CHOP. It was a combination of Cyclophosphamide (Cytoxan), Doxorubicin, Vincristine and Prednisone. Why it is called CHOP is beyond my ability to imagine.

The purpose of chemotherapy in the treatment of cancer is to kill, in a controlled way, as much of the disease as possible. Because cancer cells grow and divide rapidly, these drugs are made to kill fast-growing cells. It is impossible to be so selective that only the cancer cells are killed and as a result there is usually some damage to healthy cells. The ones most likely to be affected are blood cells forming in the bone marrow and digestive tract, (causing nausea), reproductive system and hair follicles (causing hair loss). They can also damage cells of the heart, kidney, bladder, lungs and nervous system. This damage is known by the medical euphemism of "side effects". A partial list includes drooping eyelids, constipation, sores in the mouth, stomach cramps, joint pain, mental depression, skin rash, dizziness, confusion, agitation, hallucinations, diarrhea, bed-wetting, fever, chills and convulsions. The responses to chemotherapy vary widely, depending on the chemical agents used and in what combination, the strength given and the individual's ability to withstand them. Some physicians use the supposedly less frightening term "anti-cancer" drugs referring to chemotherapy. They are very powerful drugs and they work, not every time, but in a sufficiently high percentage that they give hope to people who would have had no chance a generation ago.

Marty was advised that if any of the drug leaked out of the I.V. and on to his skin while dripping into his body he should get help immediately because he could receive a severe burn. During one of the chemotherapy sessions a little of the drug he was receiving spilled on the floor. A nurse wiped it up using a huge quantity of paper toweling. She did it furtively, telling Marty that she would be disciplined if she was caught wiping it up without donning elaborate protective gear. It took about an hour and a half on each of three consecutive days to give him the full course of chemotherapy.

I spoke to him a few hours after his third round of chemotherapy. He was in his office. He sounded edgy.

"How're you doing, kiddo?"

"Eh, all right, I guess. So far I'm not feeling a goddamn thing. They shoot me with the chemicals. I have to waste half a day, it's uncomfortable and no results."

"Are you able to get any work done?"

"I don't know. I sit here supposedly grading papers while I play an addictive computer game. I can't stop my mind from running wild."

"Marty, why don't you find a tree to sit under and try to relax yourself?"

On the border of impatience with me, he said, "I'd rather sit in my office and make an attempt at grading papers than just wait for the chemicals to *shmeiss* me. Unless I keep myself active I obsess about the future. What happens if the chemo doesn't work? What next? Is there a next? Would they try a different mixture, a different strength or would they just give it up?"

"Are you able to just concentrate on the present and not preoccupy yourself with what may happen?" My voice was determinedly soft. Now was not the time to argue.

Marty exhaled. He was marshalling his patience. "It's easier said, Sauly. The health plan would rather not pay for a transplant, probably save $200,000 if I cooperated and just died quietly."

"Aren't they obliged to pay for it?"

"I don't know. The literature says fifty is the cutoff age. Some cases fifty-five. At fifty-eight they could say the risks outweigh the benefits or that the procedure is experimental. I don't know what I could do if they refused, and I'm trying my best not to think about it. It drains me. I'd rather think of devising ways to make it happen as soon as possible. The goddamn chemo won't cooperate yet."

There was nothing further to say. Now was not the time to ask about Vilunya or the kids or to discuss some current event. Marty wanted to be alone with his black thoughts. "Well, listen, mano, take care of yourself."

"Yeah, okay, Saul, uh, thanks for the call."

On the theory that he would be properly conditioned for the transplant by the chemotherapy he had just started, he had applied for, and had been granted, a leave of absence for the teaching year of 1992-1993. A sour little irony. If the chemotherapy was successful, he would be far too weak and sick to teach. If it didn't work, he would be healthy enough to teach but closer to death.

Marty carried this encyclopedia of potential horrors around with him all the time. He discussed them with Vilunya, with me, and maybe with some other friends, but he had to think about all of them, all the time. In addition to living his life; thinking about going to our family reunion that summer, maybe with a side trip to Washington State to go sailing, nursing his kitchen garden tomatoes along until early August harvest began, finishing his work at school, keeping up with all the activities of daily life while measuring his strength carefully, he had to be thinking strategically. He had to be thinking of how to convince his health plan to agree to pay for the transplant and anything else his case required to save his life and what precise steps to take to give him the best fighting chance.

We spoke on the telephone often over the next few months. Many of those conversations were uncomfortable for me. I had to force myself to make some of those calls. What I wanted to hear was that Marty was fatigued and puking or demonstrating some of the other symptoms that proved the chemotherapy was working. It was not working. He showed none of the symptoms nor did his counts show much of a difference. He was not being conditioned for the transplant. What would happen then? Were there other steps that could be taken to condition him? Could he have the transplant without being conditioned? How I hated that word, "conditioned." More medical euphemisms. To me, a more accurate word was "tortured."

My sketchy knowledge of the subject left me confused and worried. I had heard no talk about what alternatives could be employed if the chemotherapy didn't work. In my mind, and I think in Marty's, the next step was a frightening void.

Against that disturbing background was the ongoing quandary about where to have the transplant. Marty and Vilunya had by now looked at several transplant facilities, two in Boston and Rappeport's facility at Yale New Haven Hospital. Some transplant centers are protocol driven, which means they seek a certain population of transplantees to further research ends, perhaps to be part of a clinical trial with randomized tests. An important part of their procedure is publishing their findings. That smacked to Marty as being less important than the transplant centers in which the paramount motive was patient care.

There were also differences in patient care procedures. Some, like Yale-New Haven, maintained strict antiseptic procedures. The patient would be in a room designed to keep out infectious agents. No one would be permitted to enter without scrubbing thoroughly first. The patient could not leave the room until discharge. No books or computers or photographs or anything else that could introduce infectious agents would be admitted to the room without being sterilized first. Other transplant centers were more relaxed. Nurses, and even visitors, were allowed to enter the patient's room without donning protective gear.

This was not the first time that Marty had to think about the possibility of a bone marrow transplant. Perhaps fifteen years before, Marty's hematologist, a courtly, dignified New Englander, who had cared for him since the onset of the disease, attended a conference on leukemia. When he returned he told Marty that a grading system had been developed to describe the prognosis of the disease. It was numerical, from 1 to 5, 5 being the poorest prognosis. He told Marty that he was a 5 and that he should think about a bone marrow transplant. At the time Marty was feeling well, working hard and controlling his disease with periodic doses of chlorambucil and prednisone. Suddenly, he was hearing from his kindly, caring doctor that he was close to death. In those days bone marrow transplants were done at only a few facilities around the country and, because of the extremely high mortality rate, were done on patients who were as good as dead anyway.

Marty was panicked. All the original fears surged; he would not see his children grow up, he would leave his wife a widow, his work would remain unfinished. Vilunya stepped in with a steady hand and brought calm to the situation. She had a background in some aspects of medicine. She was a founding member of the Boston Women's Health Book Collective, which wrote, "Our Bodies, Ourselves." She also holds a masters degree in Public Health from Harvard, which she earned while their children were young. She doubted the new diagnosis from the first. After a brief period of halting indecision they both cast about in their network of contacts to try to reason through the fear. Virtually everyone they spoke to, including a friend who was a Nobel laureate in Bio-Chemistry, advised him against the transplant. I spoke to the twin transplant specialist at the Hutchinson Transplant Center at the University of Washington who agreed that it was too early to consider transplant. Marty said that, in declining the transplant he was listening to his body. He also said that he had no wish to become The Martin Diskin Memorial Wall-Hung Urinal at the University of Washington.

That episode left him with a serious problem. To be a leukemia patient of the same doctor for many years virtually guarantees that a relationship develops that is much deeper than merely a consumer and provider of services. The decisions made by the doctor literally affect the life of the patient; what kind of life he will have, how long a life. Marty always spoke of his twinkly, bowtie-wearing New Englander doctor with affection and respect. He especially liked the advice he received from him early in his disease to plan ahead, to keep planning. Marty repeated that advice often.

After the comfort of being satisfied with the years of care he had been given, suddenly the advice he was getting was dead wrong and to follow it might have resulted in his death. There was unanimity of opinion about it. His trusted doctor on the one side and everyone else on the other. Why? What had motivated him to give such advice? A speculation that had great currency among us at the time was that before he retired that doctor wanted to be associated with a path-breaking event: an identical twin bone marrow transplant for chronic lymphocytic leukemia. It had either never been done before or very few had been done world-wide. It took Marty several months before he could confront his doctor. He asked him, face to face, why he had given that advice. The doctor hung his head and couldn't answer. He retired from practice a short time after that and Marty began with a new hematologist.

Marty had decided that he wanted to be under the care of Dr. Rappeport and that meant that he had to be transplanted at New Haven. The health plan had said early in the process that if they approved a transplant they wanted it done in Boston where, presumably, they had certain discounted fee arrangements of long standing.

Dr. Wellington, Marty's lead health plan doctor and Dr. Rapperort started discussing it. The correspondence and phone calls and faxes dealt almost exclusively with mechanical matters such as tissue typing between Marty and me, Marty's past medical background, discussion of latest therapeutic techniques, timing of the transplant, sinus surgery, possible removal of Marty's spleen, and chemotherapy before the transplant. All these communications assumed that there would be a transplant, which all the planning and questioning they were doing would lead to the transplant. No one outside the health plan ever asked whether permission would be granted for the transplant. Everyone acted as if there would be one at the end of the planning period. The health plan spoke in an uncertain way about the transplant and in one early letter questioned whether the committee would approve a transplant.

Dr. Wellington deferred to the bone marrow transplant specialists who are considered the high wire specialists of hematology. He referred to himself as the "last and least of several wise hematologists who have worked with Professor Diskin."

There was no result after the full four rounds of chemotherapy. We believed that the health plan would not have authorized the chemotherapy without considering it a possible step toward the transplant. Our optimistic chronology was that the transplant, after the successful chemotherapy, would take place that fall of 1992. Unless the chemotherapy produced a remission, his poor prognosis would give the committee the reason to deny him.

Arline and I visited Marty and Vilunya in late June, a couple of weeks after his second round of chemotherapy. Marty was unchanged from the time I saw him last, except that he moved a little more slowly and deliberately. Friends had to help till and plant his vegetable garden. Seeing the garden go in pleased him greatly. It was the continuation of normalcy. He would survey the garden every day, give it a little water if a patch here or there looked dry to him. He had gotten some color from being outdoors and aside from being slightly gaunt, which was not unbecoming to him, he looked pretty good. Marty and Vilunya had decided to come to the family reunion on the west coast and combine it with a visit to a friend in Seattle. What the hell. If the chemotherapy was not making him sick he might as well enjoy the summer.

The doctors discussed the use of the drug fludarabine monophosphate, newly approved by the Food and Drug Administration. An experimental drug. There was a certain thrill to the thought, a vulgar, Hollywood sound to it. The heroic moment at the end of the drama, the worthy protagonist saved by the forces of good. On the other hand, soberly thought through, it was also clear that the traditional, the well understood and widely practiced methods were just not working.

Summer was on us in Phoenix and the inhuman heat was searing the remaining energy out of me. Business was poor. The land market had not begun to recover from the terrible erosion of value it had suffered in the late eighties. Whereas, in perhaps 1986 or 1987, I was certain that I could have retired and lived quite comfortably on investments, as the market deteriorated I questioned that certainty. I hadn't earned any money in several years. We were living on investments and, while that was essentially enough to sustain us, a significant fraction of that income was shaky. I was not thinking clearly. I longed to be away from my daily round and I wanted a respite from obsessing about Marty. I also wanted to see him again, in August, on the California coast, near Santa Barbara, where the sea breezes would blow cool and where most of our extended family would gather for a few days.

Our mother did not know that the transplant was being planned or even talked about. She had been told that Marty had leukemia some ten years before, when our father was still alive. I had arranged to meet Marty in Los Angeles on his way back from a Central American trip for the purpose of telling them both. He had known about his leukemia by then for ten years and was sufficiently at ease with the future that he knew he could tell them about it without conveying an atmosphere of crisis. We arranged to have dinner with them in their shabby apartment in a Yiddish and Russian speaking neighborhood.

After the dinner of gray potroast and lifeless vegetables, we cleared the table and Marty announced that he had something to tell them. They both became anxiously attentive, sensing bad news. In soft, patient, professorial, evenly modulated tones, Marty told them the history of his illness. Without drama, trying to reduce the impact, he waited until the very end of his narrative before he used the word leukemia. They both gasped. Mom sat rooted in her chair sobbing softly, twisting her handkerchief and looking bewildered. Dad left the table abruptly and went to the other room to cry.

He returned shortly and the questions began. Marty answered, permitting them to interrupt freely. At some moment in the discussion our father said, almost to himself, "Why couldn't it be me?" It was exactly what he told Marty and Vilunya years before after the death of their baby. It fell on the ear like biblical thunder because there was no doubt that he meant it. A year or so later he died of a stroke at the age of 86.

And now we were all sitting in our mother's condominium in Los Angeles where we had arranged to meet before the family reunion to tell her about the transplant. She had bought the condominium shortly after our father's death. Several blocks from their apartment, the condominium was something she had wanted for a long time. It was larger and had a tiny balcony that she filled with plants. The new carpeting and faux elegant furniture in a three story, security building, with an elevator made her feel accomplished, arrived, in the proper atmosphere to reign as matriarch.

Mom was beaming as she surveyed her three sons (our younger brother, Phil, who lives in Los Angeles, had joined us), Vilunya and Leah and Aaron, sitting in her living room after breakfast. Everyone was bulging with smoked and pickled fish and sharp cheeses. The balcony window was open and a muscular breeze blew into the room shaking the leaves and gently rocking the limbs of the formidable sycamore tree looming outside. Marty was sitting on the French provincial couch, his arm on the back and, bridging Vilunya, was lightly touching mother's shoulder. Quiet had fallen on the room, partly in physical appreciation of the gluttonous breakfast just completed and partly to avoid the subject we had come to discuss with mother. I looked out the open window, beyond the sycamore, out to the cobalt sky daubed with clouds so white the eye hurt, and thought of Lake Hiawatha the summer of 1943 when Marty and I were nine years old.

I don't think Lake Hiawatha was an actual place on a map then. I believe it was a real estate development, a summer colony. The lake was a mile or so away from the bungalow we rented. It was a summer of milestones, each of which, after all these years, is still sweet in memory. Phil, was 14 months old and it was there he took his first steps.

Our mother was in her early thirties. She was strong and confident and eager to show off her physical abilities. She would do cartwheels and hold a handstand with her feet balancing against a wall. Snapshots taken in the late twenties and early thirties showed her in groups of young men and women, arms draped over each others shoulders. The eager, wild-haired immigrant faces with guileless, joyful looks peered at the camera, bedecked in striped two piece men's bathing suits and the women's one piece suits of the time. There was Rhoda, the Americanized Rachel, our mother, happy in the shape and performance of her youthful body, happy to be one of the group, happy to be in America. We were familiar with the stories she told us of her physical prowess as a young girl in Russia. But mostly, her stories of Russia were about the poverty and hunger she saw and experienced, about the deaths of playmates from starvation and disease, about the cruelty toward the Jews in the Moldavanka, the Odessa slum in which she lived. Every once in a while she told a story of a triumph, usually involving her athletic skill, in which she beat boys at sporting contests. We were raised on those stories. We knew them all, the stories of atrocities and of triumph. The stories were usually told to us to illustrate how much we had in contrast to what she had when she was our age, and how spoiled it had made us. We resented those stories and were bored by them, and when we showed that we were bored or impatient, which we did at times to be deliberately disrespectful, she would wallop us with uncontrolled fury and without warning.

Only as an adult did I form the image of our mother in the midst of the depressing, fear-ridden, urban prison she lived in as a child, laughing her thrown back redheaded laugh, racing, jumping rope, throwing a ball, exuberantly flexing her young muscles and daring the world, the Cossacks, the Czar, to stifle her. Her surroundings did not depress her. She did not reflect on them. She reflected on nothing. Reflection frustrated and threatened her. Smashing down the door was her style.

She was squarely built, solid and powerful. Her henna-enhanced hair framed her summer freckled face, softening somewhat the thrust of her bulbous nose. Her eyes glowed with the pleasure of physical activity. She would draw deeply on her cigarette, holding it with ostentatious confidence, like a woodman hefting a felling ax.

That summer Marty and I walked to the lake by ourselves and there, watching the big boys, learned to fish with a handline. Baiting our hooks with doughballs and the occasional worm we dug, we caught sunfish, bass, pickerel and carp. We weren't allowed to go in the water beyond our waist without our mother's supervision. The lake was really a large pond, probably man-made, with a small sand beach, both of which must have been created as amenities to attract buyers and renters for the lots and bungalows nearby. In the middle of the lake, a great distance for a little boy was a raft, a wooden island of fulfillment for Marty and me, clearly beyond our attainment.

We were good swimmers, comfortable in the water. One day our mother swam with us and after a few strokes beyond where our feet could touch bottom, told us we were going to the raft. Apprehensive but excited, Marty and I set out, stroking alongside Mommy. After a long time and great exertion, the raft was still far out of reach, the shore even further. Panic gave way to profound fatigue. We cried for help, despairing of ever reaching the raft. Mommy came alongside of first one and then the other and pinched us painfully on the thigh, on the back, on the arm. She did it again and again, deaf to our pleas. We were soon alongside the raft, looming much larger up close than from the shore. With our last energy we mounted the bobbing haven and fell down in the sun, exhausted, to rest. We lay on the raft, contented, proud of our achievement, letting the sun bake energy back into our scrawny bodies. Swimming back was easier.

Near our bungalow was a large meadow that gave way to what must have been a remnant of original forest. At the edge of the meadow, close to the wood, was a wild pear tree of gargantuan proportion. We climbed into it, scrambling high in its branches, from stout limbs to thinner ones, barely thick enough to hold our weight and swaying in the invigorated breeze. From that perch we could look up 20 feet or more into the crown of the tree and out at a countryside without end. High in the tree was our land of skywalkers, of airplane pilots, of acrobats, of muscled, handsome, heroes.

At least Marty and I were sure that Sydell thought so, who stared up at us from the ground with admiration. Sydell was our age but possessed of a precocity that frightened and attracted us. She flirted with us both and tantalized us with suggestions that we did not specifically understand, but believed were descriptions of pleasurable activity. As the summer progressed the titillation increased. In the dim light of a small enclosed shed we exposed ourselves. We feasted on the sight of her hairless vagina, almost obscured by her protruding, baby belly and she saw our tiny penises and undescended testicles. At the end of the summer, with only a few days remaining, she proposed an escalation of our activities. In our grotto of sensual exploration we agreed to touch the object of our ardent interest. She touched us softly, first one and then the other with one hand and, almost as quickly, withdrew. I bunched my fingers together as if believing that the feeling would be concentrated in my fingertips and, when I was satisfied that my fingers were properly arranged, gently brushed her soft, sweet cleft. And then we left the shed and resumed play on the grass near the the front door of the house so that we could also keep an eye on Phil.

Phil was a strikingly good looking baby. His friendly, curious, alert face drew people to him, cooing and petting. He loved the attention and rewarded strangers with delightful antics. One such admiring stranger took a series of photographs of him on the beach. In an anatomically impossible pose, Phil has his black-curled head in the sand and his ample bottom solidly rooted in the sand, his rolls of smooth skinned fat giving emphasis to his contorted pose. He showed no inclination to stand upright, much less to walk. If an adult hoisted him to his feet to encourage a step or two he responded by accentuating the gravitational pull toward earth and plopping down with decisiveness. His customary body position was sitting, his upper body moving actively, his beautiful face alert and engaging, his lower body still, solid and unmoving.

One day he got to his feet and walked away. No groping up the leg of a chair or even vigorous crawling. No preamble, no hint. Marty and I were aware of his absence only after our mother inquired about him. We were playing on the tiny survived patch of trampled grass in front of the bungalow where Phil was supposedly sitting under our watchful eye. We all looked down the dirt road in front of the bungalow and perhaps fifty yards away Phil was receding from sight. He had severed the adhesions that bound his backside to the earth and he was moving to a different climate. His legs were chugging rhythmically with determined cadence, balancing his upper body, listing perilously, now to port, then to starboard, his chubby hands articulating wildly at the wrists. His hands were lee boards, seeking resistance in the sea of air he was navigating and successfully preventing his plump boat from capsizing. We ran after him, gleefully exhorting him to return and, failing to persuade him to alter his course, took him by the hands, Marty on one side and myself on the other and steered him around toward home. He looked at us with a wondrous smile, pleased beyond expression at his accomplishment and glad for the escort of his big brothers. He came with us willingly, exulting in his newly risen status.

With barely a preamble, Marty began telling Mom about the transplant. We had all lived with it for a very long time, and, at age 58, both Marty and I had ample evidence of our own mortality aside from the fact of leukemia. Although the transplant was a frighteningly large step, it could not have been a great surprise to anyone but mother. She sat dumbly, expressionless. When Marty was finished with his explanation she asked him what it meant. She wanted to know, although couldn't say it, whether Marty would die. She wept inaudibly during the discussion, while from time to time, Vilunya or Leah or Marty embraced and caressed her. Phil, who had been a medic during his army service, made soothing, authoritative statements to reassure her. It was obvious that mother did not want to hear this news. She wished Marty's disease, this news, this talk of transplants, of medicine, of science, of death, did not exist, would be erased.

She asked me what I thought; almost as if it was a subject we could resolve with a vote. Four to two against - sorry leukemia, you lose. Her voice was heavy, distracted, distant. She could not apprehend any more of the detail, of the specifics. Although we had, in turn, given her much more assurance about the safety of the procedure and the certainty of a good outcome than any one of us felt inwardly, she was not persuaded or consoled. What she wanted was God's guarantee that she would die before Marty. She lumbered to her feet and went heavily to her bedroom to lie down while the rest of us, feeling shreds of undeserved guilt over not being able to raise Mom's lowering spirits, set out to raise our own spirits by planning the remainder of the day's activities.

We convened at a resort motel close to Santa Barbara. The sprawling single and two story buildings lay on the beach in the lee of the hills studded with oak brush, tall wild grass, and scrub pine. Beyond was the freeway, bordered by decadent, formal plantings that separated the seaside from the hills. Huge pines of fantastic shape, dangerous, almost carnivorous in aspect, menaced with evil beauty. The Mediterranean landscaping enveloping the motel grounds was common to that hospitable climate; air softer and milder than the Mediterranean, with a sensual sea breeze that exhausts one with joy. Despite the mantle of opulence the landscaping was supposed to impart, the scattered structures of the motel looked like a slightly more modern version of the Dew Drop Inn of west Texas of the fifties. Perfect for our family, for the extended Yampolskys, my mother's tribe. Ivan, one of the young cousins, called it The Yamclan.

Of the six Yampolsky children of Shifra and Mendel who survived childhood, four came to the U.S. starting from about 1906, in the first wave, to 1925, when our mother came, after the First World War and the Russian revolution. Of those four, two were left, Rhoda, our mother and Leda, her sister. Sarah and Harry, the other two, died, each at about the age of ninety. Leda was then about 85 and our mother, about 82. Ages were somewhat approximate, all the children having been born at home and not being anxious to announce the birth of a new Jew in czarist Russia. Two brothers, Abram and Yossif, whom the family called Yoska, believers in the October revolution, stayed in Russia, both of them volunteering to work building Magnitagorsk, a strategic city in the foothills of the Urals, in 1930. There they spent their lives, pioneers in a threatening wilderness, sharing the company of criminals, political undesirables and others like themselves, foreigners in their native and beloved land. Because they were Jews they were thought less of than the criminals who were forcibly transported to that wild country to build the city. A significant number of the people who built Magnitagorsk died of the cold, of disease, of the constant privation. Abram was killed in the second world war, "defending the motherland from the fascist beast," according to Yosif, who died peacefully in Magnitagorsk at the age of about 92.

The reunion was a great success because all the reunards energetically wished it so. Of the 31 blood relatives 12 were the young cousins, from the age of 8 to 35. The rest of us had seen each other all our lives. We were aware of the milestones in each others lives, even of those who lived in distant cities. We ranged from the early 50s to about 85. We were aware, each with his own individual, personal stab of anguish, that death was subtracting from what we had always considered our family and the additions of the next generation had not yet appeared. Gathered all together for the first time perhaps ever and seeing the evidence of our eyes; the stooping infirmities, the gray and baldness, the failing senses, we knew that we could not fend death off any more than our elders could. We were simply next.

The young cousins were a joyous sight to behold and something of an enigma to me. When we were children Marty and I had to be dragged to family gatherings. We valued the consanguinity much less than we did the comradeship of our chosen friends. These present youngsters, these pups, seemed to actually delight in each other's company. They spoke at length with each other, inquiring about current (and sometimes, past) relationships. They asked each other detailed questions, motivated by more than politeness, concerning achievements, plans for the future. They huddled and traveled in ever changing groups, laughing, making fun of the graybeards, coming close to the edge of insolence, always laughing an uproarious, sometimes marijuana-inspired laugh. They were lovely to see and they filled me with a proprietary feeling of love toward them all.

Marty was a welcome sight to the assembled family. Everyone remarked more with relief than enthusiasm, that Marty looked well. To those who asked specific questions about his condition he explained patiently what the near future would hold for him. His situation was starkly contrasted with that of Ed, a cousin by marriage, who was suffering from a brain tumor that would probably kill him in a short time. In a wheelchair, Cousin Ed also looked good and was mentally as alert as he ever had been.

He visited as much as his strength allowed, eagerly speaking to as many people as he could. He left all he spoke to with a touch of sadness. All knew it was a leave-taking.

I marveled at this strange and wondrous group as I wandered from cluster to cluster finding out about recent developments in their lives. Four generations were present. From the Ukraine and Lithuania we came, through Turkey and Danzig, to the sweatshops of New York to California, Massachusetts, Arizona, Ohio, England, Italy and Thailand and other places in between. A move of a continent every generation. From the poverty and oppression of village and ghetto we were now PhDs, businessmen, a literary agent, an inventor, actors, an editor, travelers of the world and samplers of its delights, well seized of our rights, despised no longer and quite confident in our place in the newest of our lands.

Marty did the same as the rest of us, walked around, stopped to talk to family members, had a coffee here with a group of three or four, a soda pop there with several more. He listened and observed more than he usually did. He evinced curiosity in a way similar to our father who would become fascinated by things that to us as kids usually were commonplace or boring: a customized license plate, a kitchen device he had never seen, a cloud formation. He had to know how it functioned or what it was. He asked questions about it, as much to himself as to anyone nearby.

I was playing tennis, alternating between singles with my son-in-law and doubles with a cousin and his wife, when I could feel Marty's stare from outside the fence enclosing the courts. He had Dad's smile of appreciation and curiosity as he watched me play tennis for the first time. What was that boy from Crown Heights in Brooklyn doing playing tennis? In Santa Barbara, California, no less. And really playing, not fooling around or pretending. We smiled at each other, a smile of unbounded pleasure and appreciation at the scene. What surged through my mind was the picture of Marty ice skating, something he did in frozen ponds in Massachusetts. I had never seen him do it and I didn't know how to ice skate myself. Someday, I would see him ice skate and maybe would try it myself.

We had meals together, we arranged tennis matches, we walked along the beach, looking out at the Channel Islands and the oil rigs. We held the old ones steady as we walked, we held the soft, sweet hands of the youngest ones, we cried at sad remembrances and laughed till we ached. We had a banquet and made speeches and passed around old photographs. We were expansive and we were nostalgic. All in three days. And then it was over. We repaired to a nearby Italian restaurant just before departing to our respective homes. We ate outdoors, under a fake grape arbor at a table without end. When we were finally finished, standing outside the restaurant, at what should have been a perfunctory round of good-byes, Sharon, my youngest daughter, hugging and kissing her uncle Marty, realized what awful uncertainty lay in front of him, and still in the embrace, began to quiver and sob. Her thin body trembled as she wept without restraint. Most of the rest of us, unable any longer to avoid the thought that this would certainly be the last time a group of our family this complete could ever again be assembled, choked and sniffled and wept softly. We were standing in a loose circle in the parking lot. As if by direction, we each scanned the circle, looked at the others one more time and separated, each to his car, and left.

In mid-September Arline and I loaded up the car and drove to Telluride in southwestern Colorado. We had rented a condominium for two weeks. Marty had agreed to join us for a week. Vilunya couldn't come because she was away on a trip in connection with her folk art business she had put off for some time because of the uncertainty of Marty's health.

The anticipation of that trip always fills me with nervous joy and the morning we set out I become a child, thrilling to the expectation of the great prize I am about to be given. The several hours between Phoenix and Flagstaff, where we have lunch, is given to remembering mountains, meadows, monuments, rivers, washes, vegetation, place names. Big Bug Creek, the Agua Fria, Horsethief Basin, the Verde River, Montezuma's Castle and finally, as the desert gives way slowly to the scrub, side oak and juniper, and as the climb begins beyond the Sedona turnoff, the Verde Valley receding behind and below, the air lightens and smells sweeter, the growth thickens and the views become shorter, until, in one clearly identifiable instant, the labor of the engine, the appearance of the tall pines and the looming San Francisco peaks announce the mountains. Beyond the Mormon Lake turnoff the dominant vegetation is the Ponderosa Pine and the year round snow covered peaks steer you straight into Flagstaff.

After lunch we head northeast across the Navajo reservation toward Southwestern Colorado. The traffic thins out as does the vegetation and as you approach the reservation the sun reflected off the bald earth stabs the eye. The views expand to the horizon in places and the settlements and other signs of human habitation become sparse. From Tuba City to Teec Nos Pos, with the exception of a trading post or two, open sometimes, there are few places to stop to buy a soda pop or gasoline. We are prepared, with sufficient water and food, should we break down. We have made this trip before.

I settle down for the several hour journey through the heart of the reservation, listening to the engine and watching the countryside slip by. The full palette of color forces the eye to adjust to the camouflaged perception of depth and distance. The color changes, but subtly, as if pigment is slowly added to what the eye and brain has understood to be reddish color until purple seems to be what is being seen. A muddy brown changes imperceptibly to a bright silver, ocher becomes magenta and vermillion. The effect is varied; from comforting to perplexing. The steady, comforting, incessant sound of the engine, accompanies the low-hilled, undulating countryside. The landscape is suggestive of a reclining nude; wind-eroded gentle curves of the striated, sandstone Modiglianis. Points of reference become lost. There are no mountains except distantly suggested, no rivers to cross, almost no traffic, only the occasional signs with place names that resonate with sacredness. We are stationary. The thrumming sound is the gear that frictionlessly pulls the countryside past our observation machine. Our conversation dies out. We sit and watch and think.

I wonder how Marty will be when I see him or if he will come at all. He began the Fludarabine treatment as soon as he returned to Massachusetts after the reunion. He was to have the second treatment just a few days before we were to leave for Telluride. Doctor Wellington tried to frighten him into canceling the trip by describing the dire consequences of getting ill in Colorado. If he should develop an infection with a high fever (over 101) and "if it got into the blood," it could be very dangerous. There might not even be time to go back to Boston. He might have to be hospitalized in Denver for weeks. Marty was downhearted and anxious. He told me in a phone call several days before we were to leave for Telluride that he decided, finally, to let his physical condition determine whether he would make the trip.

The reason for the Fludaribine treatment was to try to achieve the results that were not able to be achieved in the chemotherapy the previous spring. If the Fludaribine were to lower his tumor burden, that is, reduce the white count dramatically and greatly lower the number and proportion of leukemic cells in his blood, they could proceed shortly thereafter with the transplant He told me he felt weak.

Arline and I stayed the night in a dumpy motel on the banks of the Dolores River in the southwestern corner of Colorado, above Cortez, the beginning of the climb into the high mountains. At about 7,000 feet the slight nip to the air in the daytime turned to cold as soon as the sun went down. After dinner and a stroll to unkink after the day of driving we got into the bed which occupied most of the room and used all the covers to stay warm. I lay in the bed feeling the heat of our bodies contained by the blankets spread luxuriantly over us and excitedly thought of driving over Lizard Head Pass the next day and hoped it would not snow, at least not hard enough to close the pass.

The sixty-odd miles from Dolores to Telluride takes about two hours. The road is narrow and in places there is little or no shoulder. Along the way there is much to savor. It is a stretch of road that graphically portrays the change in climate and geography from the friendly, wooded beginnings of the alpine forest and meadow to the survival threatening wildness of the naked upthrusted peaks high above the tree line where violent storms strike with little warning and the wind cuts at you year round, assaulting the unprotected places on your body. The introduction to this area is a long river valley that narrows as it climbs, revealing hay fields on the lee side of the river that twists and cuts its way through the green sea. When it is warm enough to open the window the perfume of the alfalfa, especially soon after it is cut, mingled with the smell of the pine woods, excites my senses. I make huge, graceful mental fly rod casts at every turn in the road I am able to see the river. Each of these results in delicate presentations to the three pound trout breaking the water to strike my fly. I play it, feeling the line tighten, set the hook and, with satisfaction, confirm the weight of the fish all in the microsecond or two before I follow the curve of the road that takes me out of sight of the river. I watch for raptors eyeing prey from on high. I try to spot wolverines or bears prowling through the woods looking for a meal.

Telluride is a resort town nestled in a deadend valley at 8,500 feet, surrounded by towering, jagged peaks of over 13,000 feet. It had been a prosperous mining town in the late nineteenth century that was reborn in recent times as a chic ski-resort town. Its buildings are restored original or faux Victorians amid many condominiums. The main street is packed with restaurants, clothing and sporting good stores, bars and establishments existing to sell "authentic" experiences or mementoes to well-heeled tourists. The San Miguel River, a decent trout stream in places, flows through the town. A smart and successful place, it is a town designed for the visitor to engage in pleasurable activities, and because it's pristine surroundings and clean, bracing air, to feel righteous at the task.

We had been there before a few times and felt like we knew the town. There were even a couple of people who remembered us from prior visits. Because we don't ski, the summer is the perfect time for us. Festivals and events as diverse as a small film festival to the wild mushroom convention are scheduled almost the entire summer. We have frozen out of doors, sitting on hard ground, seeing an attempt at Shakespeare as well as a Grateful Dead concert performed almost under our balcony. I was eager to begin fly fishing and walking some of the trails. I was bubbling with little boy's excitement at being back in the mountains.

Thinking of Marty was making me anxious and mildly guilty. I wondered if he would be able to withstand the elevation, whether he would undertake too much activity, whether he would have the same interest in fishing I did and, with a stab, whether the chemotherapy he had begun would make him sick and ruin our stay. Arline and I had scheduled a one day float trip on the Gunnison River. I would fish from the raft and Arline would enjoy the changing wild terrain. Marty decided against going, thinking the trip too strenuous for him.

The Telluride airport and terminal is sited on a high mesa a few miles out of the town. The views are of the world below, extending in places to the horizon. We arrived twenty minutes or so before Marty's plane was due to arrive. I paced nervously around the building until a faint growl in the eastern sky could be heard heralding the arrival of the 12-place plane from Denver. Minutes later the plane itself could be seen and we watched its long approach and landing. Then, because of the muffled public address system, we went to the wrong door entering the terminal. Minutes passed and no Marty. In a panic I ran around looking for him with no success. Finally, running out the door to the graveled parking lot where I thought he might have gone thinking we had not yet shown up to meet him I almost stumbled over him. He was sitting on his bag, slumped and tired-looking, but with a broad smile signifying his relief that his journey was over and a certain devilish enjoyment at my consternation over misplacing him for a few minutes.

Arline and I were noticeably conscious of Marty's fragility and our solicitude must have struck him. He told us immediately that we were not to interrupt our activities nor change our schedule because of his visit. When he needed to, he told us, he would rest or nap as his spirits and his level of strength dictated. He seemed in good enough shape to me, his energy level high considering the length and duration of the trip. By the next morning he had gotten over the effects of the trip and we were planning a few hours fishing on the San Miguel.

Marty moved ploddingly. His speech was measured, solemn. I thought about it perfunctorily, deciding that it was the remnants of the trip fatigue. The three of us walked a nearby trail together. Marty kept up with no strain. In fact, the elevation, well over 10,000 feet, seemed to affect him less than it did me. The fishing tired him and he was very tentative about wading in the river. I took pleasure in instructing him and he accepted it with interested attention. It was in contrast, I thought, to the days of our childhood when the only important thing about such an occasion would have been to see who could catch the first or most fish and gain the standing to be able to taunt the other one unmercifully. I watched him concentrating on his fishing, making delicate casts and I felt a swell of tearful love for him, a feeling closely akin to what I would have felt for a child of mine who had just been hurt. He caught a fish and we both exploded with joy, undoubtedly frightening the nearby fish. We feasted on trout and wine that night.

The next morning Marty said he would pass up the walk that had become our morning custom. I decided to stay behind with him and Arline went by herself. The day was overcast and the view from the window leading out to a small balcony was dramatically enhanced by the filtered light. We puttered around a bit, silently clearing the breakfast dishes and settled finally on the generic, rental-property couches arranged perpendicular to each other facing a large television set. Marty wanted to talk. He made himself comfortable as I tensed, instinctively, to listen.

"Since I saw you last and probably before then, I have been depressed."

"Just feeling bad, or blue, or really depressed, as in needing help depressed?" I was uneasy.

Marty looked away from me. He had a story to tell me. "I think clinically depressed is accurate to say. I can't seem to concentrate on much of anything. If I try to read I fall asleep in no time. I want to sleep a lot. I feel myself getting sour, nothing pleases me. I feel needy. I want Vilunya to minister to me, to take care of me when I need it."

"What's wrong with that? You're sick and you're going to need help and understanding. Why shouldn't Vilunya help you? Doesn't she want to?"

"Yeah, she wants to help me. She does all that is realistic for me to expect. You know me. I want more than is realistic. It also seems to me that she has retreated a little into her business so she doesn't have to face my lousy situation. It scares the hell out of her, the thought of my dying. Everything is up in the air now. The goddamned Fludarabine isn't working. If it doesn't do the job I don't know what the hell will happen next, whether I can even have the transplant."

"What does the health care plan doctor say? Or Rappeport?"

"I don't know any more. It's all I can do to get one piece of information straight at a time when I talk to those guys. All kinds of things are mentioned. More chemotherapy, maybe different drugs, maybe a splenectomy. For Christ's sake, I don't even know yet whether the health plan will authorize the expense of the transplant or if they will whether they'll let me use Rappeport or make me use one of the places they are aligned with."

We sat in silence for a while. Marty was not finished. There was more on his mind, something darker and more frightening.

"Look, Marty, do you think you could use some shrinkage or some counseling, some professional to talk to about this?"

"You know, Sauly, I don't even know whether I want to go through with what lies ahead," he said heavily, his voice steady, but laden with despair, with surrender. "I'm wondering if it wouldn't be better if I just died. Better for everyone around me, better for me."

Neither one of us could talk any more at that point. Tears leaked out of our eyes. I looked out the window at the giant leaden slag heap to the east and the Bridal Veil Falls rising above it in the distance. I felt cold and useless.

"Do you ever think about my death?"

"Yes," I said flatly.

"Do you flesh the scenes out with dialogue, with other people, like at my memorial? Do you imagine the particulars?"

I told him I didn't think about it with such specificity. I lied to him. I had thought a lot about Marty's death, mostly about what it would do to me. I pictured the moment I would be aware of his death and feared what my reaction would be. The scenes were always awful. The knowledge would fell me. A giant machete slashing me from shoulder to midsection, a hot poker pain in my stomach, a blacking out. Those images were easy to cast away, but what would always begin to form as I rid myself of them was the thought, the beginning of a question that frightened me so I would stifle it before it could find voice in my mind: when Marty dies, will I die, too?

I also imagined myself at his funeral service, addressing the assembled group of people. I spoke only because I was pressured into it by Marty.

He loved such public occasions and he knew I did not. I was angry that I had succumbed and resentful that I had to go through with it. I told the assembly that I was not going to hold forth about Marty's accomplishments or the contributions he made in his lifetime or the sterling person he was. I would simply say that my sorrow was private, that I loved my brother and he was no more. I would have wanted to say that nobody there could understand my grief, but I didn't.

We cried a little as we talked. Not long, wracking sobs or gushers but enough so that our eyes were wet and swollen and, from time to time, our speech silenced by tears. After a time Marty said it would be harder on me if he died first. I understood completely, but just to test the twin understanding after all these years of being apart, I said to him, "Because if you died first I would have all those years to live without you, but if I died first it would be the end of the twins because without the transplant you would soon follow." He nodded in agreement.

The day broke in my solar plexus with the rivet gun sound of the alarm clock. My eyes clanged open with the immediate boyish anticipation of a fishing day as well as the tiniest apprehension that maybe the alarm clock had malfunctioned and it was really too late. No, the time was right, 4:30 AM, plenty of time to arise, complete all morning ablutions and drive with Fred and his friend Phil to Montrose, where we were to be picked up by the outfitter's bus and taken to the Gunnison River to spend the day drifting some 14 miles through wild country and, more importantly to me, through great trout water.

I was completely ready at least 15 minutes before we had to meet Fred, my friend and business associate who, with his wife and another couple, was also vacationing in Telluride. All my fishing gear, twice checked the night before, was neatly stacked at the door. I had made a thermos of coffee and I took a cup out on the balcony, in the chill, pre-dawn air. I felt mildly apprehensive about Arline joining us. She is not physically robust or agile. The outfitters had told us that there would only be one or two rapids worthy of the name.

I didn't want to have to look after Arline, especially if it would impede my fishing in any way. I wanted complete freedom to behave like an idiot if I wanted, to carry on with the other fishermen without fear of ridicule or criticism. I wanted, and felt I needed, a day with no responsibility and, I realized with a pang, that also meant a day without thinking about Marty constantly. The cold sting of air in my chest inflated me with the wonderful potential of the day to come, and I brushed aside my qualms. Arline was very eager to join us. She loves to be on water and she has a profound appreciation of wild scenic beauty. I knew she was going to love the whole day and carry away a bright memory.

Turning my back to the dull light coming out of the apartment I stared out into the blackness. I could see nothing yet, but looking to the east out past the beaver pond below, in the direction of the jagged peaks of the San Juans rising from Imogene Pass, I searched for the first light which, according to my estimate, had to appear soon. Not distracted by either the slapping sounds of the beaver's tails or the occasional sip of coffee, I stared intently into the dark. Gradually, the smallest difference in gradation appeared. Black and slightly less black. Not even gray yet. Whether the eye or the brain first apprehended it the difference slowly became discernible. It was as if there was the tiniest backlighting of the looming mountain. Now grays appeared and became lighter, insinuating the outline of the peaks. Nascent light appeared in different parts of the nightscape, as from a distant nebula, diffuse and eery, gave contrast to the slag piles in the foreground. And then, from the distant sky, the very first streaks of mauve stealing softly across the peaks, stabbing into the slopes and the valley below, brought promise of illumination to the day. My heart swelled, my spirit felt a chorus of hundreds of voices, accompanied by a full symphony orchestra singing a hymn of optimism, of confidence that the new day would bring a day of thrilling sights and unforgettable fishing.

The gear tucked securely away, the four of us set out for the Gunnison; Fred, Phil, Arline and I. In deference to Arline the conversation was more adult than it would have been and the kidding between Fred and Phil and me somewhat softer. Much attention was given to the coffee, the pouring and passing around of cups, presided over by Arline. With the evolving sunrise backlighting us, we made our way to Montrose, where, by now in full daylight, we waited at a dingy convenience market to be picked up by the outfitter's. From afar we must have looked like a group of derelicts, stamping our feet and shuffling in place to ward off the morning cold, waiting for jobs at day labor. Some derelicts, dressed in expensive sport clothing and huddling around our fishing equipment, the aggregate value of which would have made a respectable down payment on a modest house.

We introduced ourselves and exchanged greetings with the rest of the river party, a group of six or seven men who all appeared to be hardware dealers from the upper Middle West who made annual fishing trips together for the past thirty years or so. They had assembled from different locations just the day before and were still exchanging reminiscences of past fishing trips. From their talk they were serious fisherman and friends of long standing. We heard stories of trout from the San Juan and Lees Ferry, the Bighorn and the Big Hole, the Madison and the Yellowstone, of Bonefish and Permit from the Bahamas and Christmas Island. Past middle age, they seemed wholesome and solid people.

Bouncing along in the minivan I talked with one of the hardware fisherfolk about Lester Thurow's latest book about the U.S.'s international trade policy. He was from an Iowa city of about 40,000. I amused myself by my prejudiced surprise as I noted both how articulate my seatmate was and how close his views on the subject were to mine. I wished that Marty could have that experience, but I also knew that the book we were discussing was one that Marty had no interest in.

As we were loading our gear on the assigned inflatable rubber rafts and making up our rods in anticipation of the first casts of the day a vigorous rain burst upon us, a line squall that lasted fifteen minutes or so. Within a few minutes of the time it stopped a slide began on the opposite bank, bleeding a huge quantity of mud and silt into the river, staining the water an opaque brown from bank to bank. The sight produced a puzzled worry on the part of the fishermen, and from the look on the faces of the boatmen it was clear that the day's fishing was ruined. We set out anyway, the boatman agitatedly trying to decide whether to stay where we were and let the sediment settle enough to permit some fishing or to try to outrun it and hope for some luck downstream.

We drifted a while, our boatman standing between his oars reading the water, Arline sitting on the rear gunwale enjoying the scenery and I standing in the front of the raft trying to temper my disappointment by practicing casting into the muck. Arline, plumply planted on her observation perch, was smiling sweetly. She was wearing a bright red plastic poncho that covered her from neck to ankle. I smiled at her, thinking fleetingly that she didn't look too secure in her seat but reasoned that the water was calm enough so that she couldn't be disturbed. Besides, I didn't want to nag her. She looked so happy to me, smiling her little girl's smile of enjoyment at all she saw.

After I had retrieved my line and was preparing for the next cast I glanced back at Arline and saw her disappearing from sight. From the awkward way she was falling toward the bottom of the raft and the way her hands were flailing in an attempt to grasp the air I knew she had been bucked off her seat and was going down heavily. With a spark of annoyance at having to suspend my casting practice, I dropped my rod and made my way back to where she had fallen. The boatman pulled us into an eddy and fastened us to a boulder near the shore. Arline was lying in the bottom of the raft on her back. She looked at me calmly and said in a clear voice, "I've broken my shoulder." It was a look I recognized. It was the look she had when she woke me at five in the morning before the birth of our second child, our daughter Bess. Arline had dressed, showered, made up, with one hand holding her big belly and the other her small, packed suitcase, announced that we had to start driving to the hospital thirty miles away. "It's time to have a baby."

Looking at her lying on her back, almost at rest, with no panic in her demeanor, I could barely reconcile her description of what had happened. From her position she gave clear instructions about how she was to be lifted upright. Fred and I lifted her painstakingly by the life jacket. When she was upright her face twisted into a grimace of pain and her eyes began to lose their focus. I asked her if she was going to faint. She told me to hold on to her for a bit and clutching my hand, she closed her eyes and waited till the spasm of pain passed. Arline, who never complains about pain, was struggling to hold on to consciousness. Now I knew how badly she was hurt.

It was late mornng. We were supposed to float down the river to the point of debarkation where Fred's car, driven by the outfitter's men, was waiting for us. It was expected that we would finish the trip at around seven in the evening. We were too far downriver to row upstream to the beginning point. The outfitter had no radio with him to call for a helicopter and, apparently, no painkiller in a medicine kit.

After receiving assurance that the rapids were all too small to throw us about it was decided to start rowing downriver as fast as possible and drive to the emergency room of a rural hospital some twenty miles away. Arline would sit on a box lashed to the raft frame in the middle of the boat, back-to-back with the boatman. He would be facing forward, Arline to the rear. After several tries Arline manuevered her arm into the least painful position where we bound it as tight to her body as she could stand with assorted bits of clothing. I then sat at a right angle to her, bracing her with my knees and wrapping my arms around her, pressing her gently against my chest: a sort of human splint.

That is how we rode down the river for almost five hours. Arline drifted in and out of full consciousness, falling into a dreamy, semi-aware state from time to time. Several times we hit large rocks and she was jolted strongly. Aside from the deep groans those stabs of pain produced she never complained. After the first few minutes I realized how difficult it was for her to even talk and I stopped trying to engage her, content to let her state of shock insulate her from the pain. Once the boatman failed to pull us out of the way of a partially submerged rock and one side of the raft caught on it as the other gunwale rose out of the water, threatening to swamp or capsize us. At the last minute the current freed us from the rock and the boat righted itself while I cursed the boatman's lack of skill. I was grateful that Arline was deep in her state and barely aware of what had happened.

When Arline seemed peacefully asleep, her face looked relaxed, as if contemplating the natural beauty floating past her. She looked beautiful to me in those moments and I prayed that there would be no storm or rapids or anything to give her pain. I scanned the one shore I could see and the sky beyond for a glimpse of wildlife. Except for a hawk and several buzzards all I saw was the semi-arid bank. A time or two I observed, with mixed feelings that the water had cleared and I mentally made casts in the direction of good trout holding places.

It was a very long day. We had to visit two hospitals, one that did the x-raying, and when the results showed a severe break of the Humerus and a formidable dislocation of the shoulder, finally administered painkillers to Arline. We had to find a second hospital where an orthopedist was on call who was competent to set and cast Arline's arm and shoulder.

We arrived back in Telluride at about one in the morning. Fred stayed with us all the time, helping in his sure and unobtrusive way. Arline was exhausted, and with the help of the painkilling drugs she had been given, fell asleep immediately.

The next morning it was possible to see the damage done to Arline. Her face was haggard, etched by black lines of fear and pain. She would have to determine what she could do for herself and which things required my help and she set about that task in her careful and methodical way, reassuring herself at every step. Her upper arm, traumatized and discolored, was swelling out of the cast. Our plan was to leave Telluride in three days time. I tried to persuade Arline to fly home. I would drive home with all our luggage. She wouldn't hear of it. My anxiety was over the pain she would feel bouncing for nine or ten hours in the car. She countered that the painkillers would keep her asleep for most of the way.

Marty bade us farewell as I slowly backed the jeep out of the parking lot. Arline was reassuring everyone with her smile and waved feebly with her uncasted arm. Marty's face was creased with worry for Arline.

In the middle of the Navajo reservation fatigue overwhelmed me. Arline spotted the symptoms and urged me to pull over to rest or sleep for a while. When I finally agreed I looked, mile after mile, for some patch of shade. Unable to stay awake any longer I pulled on to the shoulder and napped for fifteen or twenty minutes while Arline patiently waited in the boiling heat. The rest of the trip went smoothly, if slowly. No flat tires, no mechanical problems. Arline checked frequently on my alertness and I on her comfort. Speaking softly to each other, sculpting the moments with our words to create a haven of ease and safety within our crowded, hastily loaded car, we carefully made our descent to the desert and home.

SURGERY

When Marty returned to Massachusetts and he and Vilunya met with Doctor Wellington, he was greeted by the worst of news. The Fludarabine therapy had not worked at all and that it would be discontinued immediately. Marty knew the Fludarabine had proved useless but he was shaken by the flat, declarative way it was said. Doctor Wellington then told him that the splenectomy would have to be done. He said, matter-of-factly, that Marty should make arrangements with the appropriate surgeon in the health plan to see about having his spleen removed. The new schedule was to have the splenectomy in late October and, after recovery, probably in late November, to begin aggressive chemotherapy using a combination of drugs know as EDAP. Assuming everything went well, the transplant could be in February of 1993. Vilunya asked about Marty's weight loss and the doctor assured her that there was nothing to worry about; it was merely muscle mass that Marty was losing.

The news was devastating to both Marty and Vilunya. Especially hard for Marty to bear was the offhand comment about losing his muscle mass. We didn't discuss it but we both had always been proud of our bodies. Skinny as boys, we always had a secret pleasure in believing that we were stronger than we looked, that even as we grew older our muscles could respond like those of much younger men. The loss of muscle mass may have been "mere" to the doctor. To us it was the frontier between middle age and the descent to hollow-cheeked, empty, debilitating old age. Winter was gathering its muscle and I pictured Marty and Vilunya stepping outside the medical building after the meeting, facing the chill wind under the threatening, slate sky and feeling older and frailer than before the meeting. In my innards I knew it was an exaggeration. Vilunya probably grabbed his arm tightly, pointedly seeking his protection against the wind and cheerily suggested that they go to a nearby shop that she knew had wonderful coffee and a certain delectable baked good.

Although splenectomy had been discussed in the past, it had been a vague and distant thought until now. Marty's spleen was huge. It bulged from his abdomen noticeably. Removing it was a serious operation. The reasons for doing so seemed murky to us all. The doctors told us that it might give the chemotherapy a better chance of working. That was the great hope. The literature suggested that hemoglobin and platelet counts often increase after splenectomy. The spleen is an active organ, a scavenger, hunting for damaged or diseased cells to destroy. It is also commonly a major site of leukemia. When the spleen enlarges rapidly, it is a strong indication that cells are replicating rapidly. If that is so, the removal of the spleen lessens the amount of disease the chemotherapy has to attack. It is called debulking. The several things I read about splenectomy and the two doctors I spoke to about it all had an uncertainty in their comments. I concluded that at this stage in Marty's illness, after trying various things that did not work, splenectomy was simply the next thing on the list. The last thing, I believed.

An ominous note in the reading I had done, one which I did not discuss with Marty, was that the mortality rate may approach 10 percent "if the procedure is done late in the course of the disease." I did not want to think about what "late in the disease" meant in relation to Marty. In any event, there did not seem to be any choice.

Marty had much to do and little time in which to accomplish it. He was at the nadir of physical and psychological strength. The first thing he did was to make an appointment with a psychiatrist specializing in oncological diseases. Dr. S., in Marty's recounting of the session, catalogued Marty's situation. His characterization was that Marty was required to make a number of choices without knowing which one or ones would be acceptable to his medical advisors or to the health plan. None of the alternatives were acceptable in that each involved the risk of either imminent death or setting in motion a chain of events that could lead to his death. If he did nothing, the outcome was certain: he would die. Therefore, he was confused, anxious, depressed, had insomnia. He seemed to suggest that Marty's reaction was entirely appropriate. While the doctor's sanctioning of Marty's feelings made Marty feel somewhat better, it did not alleviate the situation. The doctor told Marty that "he was the kind who raises problems."

He didn't mean that Marty had raised the problem of leukemia. He meant, and it was undeniably so, that Marty subjected the present situation, as well as other, more abstract subjects, such as politics, to microscopic analysis. What better subject to microscopically analyze than the immediate threat to one's life? What more engrossing or important subject? In any event, that was how Marty was. One session with a shrink was not going to change a life-long pattern. Marty sounded a little stronger to me after the session. He said that he felt a little better after the disappointment of hearing that the Fludarabine therapy was stopping and that he had to have the splenectomy. He declared that he would marshall his strength and concentration for the task that lay ahead. We spoke frequently on the phone, conspiring. Marty would tell me his intentions and the strategy he thought proper to employ. I would comment and make suggestions. This was not medicine we were talking about. It was negotiation, something at which I had served a long apprenticeship. The outcome of this matter was more important than any real estate deal I had ever negotiated.

Marty suspected that the chemotherapy he had been prescribed had not been aggressive enough to produce a good outcome. From various communications in which he commented about Marty's condition, his doctor was fatalistic in his description and grudging about the possibility of a bone marrow transplant being of benefit. It sounded like a cost benefit analysis in which the analysis of the data is presented to justify the conclusion already reached. The institutional bias was clear: a lot of money could be saved if they could deem Marty to be a marginal candidate for the BMT and manage him as an end-stage patient, that is, make him comfortable till he died.

That attitude and the inevitable outcome it predicted frightened and angered Marty. He wasn't going to put up with it. He was going to fight. Being treated for depression, getting weaker and battling against time, he began his campaign. The time pressure was perhaps the most urgent. Some eight months earlier he had been told that there were "perhaps months left" until his condition might change significantly. That meant that his immune system was sufficiently compromised so that an opportunistic infection - pneumonia, the old man's friend - might kill him. With winter fast approaching that likelihood was anything but remote.

The first thing to determine was that he could have the transplant in New Haven. The Health Plan told Marty they would give a definite answer soon. Marty and Vilunya went to New Haven, visited Dr. Rappeport and his staff and formally asked him to take over the management of his case. Rappeport agreed, provided Marty got the approval of his Health Plan. Marty scheduled a meeting with Doctor Wellington for the purpose of convincing him to relinquish the management of his case to Rappeport. Without his support it would be easier for the committee to refuse based on any reason that had the color of reasonableness. The easiest of these were that Marty was too old and the procedure experimental.

Throughout the country there were an increasing number of cases of medical insurers refusing to pay for procedures they called experimental. In a celebrated case in California involving an autologous transplant for breast cancer, the woman died after the procedure. The jury that heard the lawsuit brought by the women's family decided it was the delay that reduced her chances for survival. Suing to force his Health Plan to pay for the transplant was not a realistic option for Marty. His time was running out.

In the meantime he spoke to several other doctors, some related to his case, some concerned friends. So far the only surgeon the Health Plan had given him permission to speak to was a contract surgeon associated with the Health Plan who had repaired a hernia for him some years before. Even though he had never removed a very large spleen before, he agreed, almost offhandedly to do the operation. Marty was trying to learn as much as he could to be able to frame his argument to his doctor in the most knowledgeable and compelling terms. In addition to general information, though, every doctor he spoke to told him that a splenectomy was not a minor operation and that it must be performed by a surgeon with a lot of experience at removing large spleens and, in the opinion of one of the doctors Marty spoke to, an oncological surgeon.

That realization changed the goal and the strategy somewhat. Instead of fighting to have the transplant done in New Haven under the care of Rappeport and the other procedures, the splenectomy as well as subsequent chemotherapy, done locally, it was now clear that all aspects of Marty's case involved critical hematological judgments and it was crucial that all the procedures be done under Rappeport's guidance, including the splenectomy. That meant that the Health Plan would be able to use very few, if any, of its own providers. Although this made Marty's task more daunting, it seemed apparent that having Rappeport manage his case exclusively would give Marty the best chance of survival.

Marty approached the forthcoming meeting with doctor Wellington like a PHd candidate preparing for his oral exams. In addition to being as well versed as to the medical aspects of his case as many non-hematological doctors, he prepared himself very carefully to make the most persuasive case possible. We spoke often on the phone and faxed messages back and forth. We discussed the actual dialogue he would employ with Doctor Wellington. The strategy was to argue his case with crystalline logic and at the same time to make the doctor see that his life was at stake, without becoming strident or defeating him in argument. He would have to come close to imploring at times and would have to be strong to the threshold of aggressiveness at times. A tough job even if the subject was selling ladies underwear. Now it was life or death.

It came off without a hitch. Marty told Doctor Wellington that the last meeting he had with him left him shaken, and proceeded, in clear language, to recapitulate the history of his case from the beginning of the first chemotherapy to the discontinuation of the Fludarabine therapy. He quoted and paraphrased the doctor who had told him that after the splenectomy, if he was still refractory to chemotherapy he would not have the BMT. No subtleties, no nuance, just cold and rigid, no BMT. He paused and then told him what it would mean not to have the BMT, not simply the fact of death but the death of a human being, of a certain Martin Diskin. He described briefly what it would mean to his family, what goals in his life he could never fulfill. He made it personal.

He then told Doctor Wellington that after he recovered from the last visit he determined to find out as much as he could about his case through reading and consulting with others. He made reference to "the literature." He mentioned a doctor he had spoken to at a nationally known cancer treatment center. He told Doctor Wellington of the importance of having a surgeon experienced with large spleens. He said that the people he spoke to told him that CLL patients being refractory to chemotherapy was not unusual and that his case was "unremarkable." He told him that the Health Plan has approved him for a BMT and Rappeport still considered him a candidate for one and that he meant to have it. He thanked him warmly, with the proper amount of studied humility, for the care he had given him up to this point and asked his help in convincing the Health Plan to let Rappeport be the manager of his case from now on and for the various procedures to be done in New Haven.

Doctor Wellington complemented him on the research he had done and enthusiastically agreed with Marty's conclusions. He said that he had brought Marty along until now and he was ready to give him into

Rappeport's care. Marty sensed that he was relieved to be retiring from what he considered a difficult case. Doctor Wellington promised he would write to Joel Rappeport as well as the Health Plan recommending what Marty wanted.

Marty left the office feeling exultant, triumphant. He had accomplished his goal. He had passed through the confrontation that he feared and dreaded and had obtained the best result. It didn't mean the matter was resolved in his favor yet but a great step had been taken. It made Marty stronger. He would need all his strength for what would follow.

Five days later Marty heard from the Health Plan that the splenectomy was approved for New Haven and that they were reasonably sure all of his care could be done there, including the bone marrow transplant. Marty immediately called Rappeport to begin the planning. A few days later all the arrangements were confirmed. He was now in the care of Dr. Rappeport, who would make all the medical decisions: what procedures would be performed, who would perform them and where. It was the middle of November.

Marty was admitted into the Yale-New Haven Hospital for the splenectomy November 30th, 1992. He spoke to me from his hospital room. He sounded good. "Sounded good" is the first observation almost everyone, including me (most of the time), makes when they speak to Marty these days. It seems to say that despite the "objective" evidence of things such as blood tests, recurrent sinus infections, constant fatigue and other indicators, all of which describe a badly weakened immune system, the surest proof that all will be well is his resolute manner and his steady voice. He was reassuring me, allaying my fears. Even as he neared the moment of his first survival test, the surgery tomorrow, I heard in his voice that he was taking care of me. I told him that Arline, after the phone call yesterday, told me that his voice sounded strong, that he sounded good. Marty assured me that he was not dissimulating, that he had thought all these things through, including thinking about death and that he was feeling strong and confident about tomorrow.

His voice had that crackle of fear around the edges. Because I am no stranger to that fear, to that inability to read the portents, I know it is sometimes harder on the onlookers than on the one who experiences it. It is proper then, that he comfort me as well as Vilunya and Leah. It also helps to distract him somewhat.

He told me that his surgeon had removed a spleen that weighed 15 kilos (33 lbs.). Marty guessed that his will weigh 10 lbs or more. People were coming into his room to get more information and do more tests. He had to leave the line. I told him, as lightheartedly as I could, that I would be thinking of him tomorrow. He reassured me again and, in a lower voice, in a tone that reached my heart, said, "I love you, Saul."

Marty and I were driving from New York City to Fort Dix, New Jersey, in the spring of 1956. I was returning him to base shortly before he was to be discharged from the Army. At that time we had not seen each other in more than two years. I had married a few months before. I had spent a couple of years before that time in California where my friends and acquaintances talked of their feelings without cease in language that was supposed to be psychologically insightful. Still in the thrall of what I had considered the healthy California openness I told Marty that I loved him. His response was curt and designed to stun me. "How do you know? We've not seen each other for a long time." It did stun me, although I recovered quickly, recognizing the preposterousness of the situation. He was finishing his army service, having just returned from Japan and now, after tasting civilian life for only a few days during his leave, he was returning to his cold barracks while I was going back to my warm bed to lie next to my young, loving, wife and all I did was talk California psychobabble.

I told Marty that I loved him very much and we hung up. He sounded good. I did feel reassured. Although I felt confident that he would withstand the surgery I struggled to avoid thinking of the time after the surgery, of the chemotherapy and whether it would be successful. Our plan was that I would come to the hospital six days from then. Because everyone harbored the hope that by the time I arrived Marty would have been discharged from the hospital and returned home to Lexington, I was scheduled to fly to Boston. If Marty was still in New Haven, I would take the train to New Haven and be with in the hospital till he was able to return home. I would accompany them and stay for a day or two in Lexington. A total time of about a week or so should do it nicely, we thought. The thought of staying longer made me somewhat nervous. It was only a little more than two months ago that Arline had broken her shoulder and she was still convalescing. Our son, Jonathan, volunteered to come from Cincinnati to stay with Arline for a week. That calmed me somewhat but I was also feeling a vague unease about having neglected business over the last few months.

I spoke to Vilunya the following day, after the surgery. She said the young woman surgeon, Doctor Ward, diminutive of stature, tweedily man tailored, said it went "super." Marty had tolerated it well and there was no sign of infection. I called the next day and Marty picked up the phone very slowly. His voice was firm, although his speech was slow. He said that he had walked around that morning, less than 24 hours after his surgery, for about 40 minutes.

He wasn't able to speak too long because he said he was bothered by nausea. He just wanted to make sure I heard his voice. I spoke to Vilunya who filled me in on everything else, which was from good to uneventful.

The thought of Marty walking around reassured me greatly. I pictured him wryly smiling his crooked smile to himself, shuffling along the corridor, pleased to be getting stronger with each step, pleased to have survived. Much different than when our father was in the hospital with a fractured skull and a worn-out heart.

In his early 80s, returning to his car in the parking lot of a high school where he was attending night classes Dad's heart stopped. He fainted and fell, fracturing his skull. Someone discovered him immediately and sent for the paramedics, who took him to a hospital where they revived him. My mother was notified and she went to the hospital and then called us. Her description of the event was on the order of a slip in the parking lot that caused him to fall and get a bump on the head, nothing life-threatening. In addition to glossing over Dad's condition, Mom did not tell us till the next day, that when she returned to her apartment very late that night she was held up at knifepoint in the garage of her apartment house. The robber told her he would not hurt her if she gave him her money. She asked him please not to hurt her as she surrendered the contents of her purse. He took what she gave him and left, almost politely.

Dad was sitting upright in his narrow, intensive care unit bed, staring fixedly straight ahead. He moved his head slowly and greeted us with enraged eyes. We approached him gingerly, awkwardly. "What a revoltin' development," he said, with as much of a twinkle as he could muster through the vise of pain. The expression delighted Dad. It came from a sitcom of the 50s with William Bendix, whose career was spent portraying gruff but lovable characters. I always thought that Dad believed the expression was quintessentially American.

The doctor told us that Dad needed a pacemaker and that the skull fracture was "formidable." He looked awful. Paled by the trauma, his olive skin looked dry and colorless against the silly, brief, hospital gown he wore.

He was a lifetime removed from the picture taken with our mother when they were married in 1930: he seated in an ornate photographer's prop chair, his back erect, his thick lips and black hair framing the look of defiant confidence shooting from his Asian, almond eyes. His right arm rested on the arm of the chair, grandly displaying a ring on his little finger, no doubt one of the first non-essential purchases of his life. Our mother sat on the left arm of the chair, poised proudly, her back straight, with athletic grace, a purposeful look about her. That, then, was our father. His high cheekbones and dark oriental features gave him a look of menace, a portrait more resembling a Kirghiz or Tajik or Turkoman tribesman, giving vent to his wild blood by whipping a lathered horse across the windblown steppe. What I saw before me in that device-filled cubicle was a tamed, cooled version of the young man of violent rages who marshaled all his will to keep from trembling with pain. Several days later he told Mom to bring his checkbook to the hospital during her next visit. When she did he wrote the remaining check to pay for the trip to Russia the following month they had been planning, to visit her recently discovered brother, Yoska. That was how he declared to Mom and the world that he was not going to die yet. He was our old father, our dad, long gone now.

Marty was not Dad, I forced myself to understand and believe. Everything was going well with Marty. He told me he walked both Thursday and Friday. Good signs. What was being awaited anxiously was the return of his digestive and excretory functions. He had urinated without a catheter and was feeling rumblings in his gut. We were full of subdued jokes about the first fart. I was planning on being there the following Monday and felt buoyant about the timing. He still sounded tired and, although his words were clear and sensible he didn't stay on the phone for long. He had a device that permitted him to receive morphine on demand. As a result he had no appreciable pain, but was a little dopey a lot of the time. Vilunya reported that the doctors were pleased with his progress. His spleen weighed close to ten pounds, about three times a normal one.

I spoke to Phil several times as well as to Mom. I heard them both characterizing the operation as a great success, as if he will be cured from leukemia when he recovers from the surgery. One thing at a time, I told myself. They have both spoken to Marty and are greatly relieved by his words and just by hearing his voice, proof that he still exists. In one of my calls to Mom she told me she was sick to her stomach. She told me she had puked till she was empty. I made her promise that if it continued, if she couldn't get to sleep or if she had extreme weakness or fever or any other severe symptom to call Phil or me or 911. Dutifully, she agreed. She attributed her illness to the emotional upset over Marty, not to flu, as I was beginning to fear. When I called the next days he said she was fine. No more puking. She was holding food down. She said this happens to her "every thirty years." "You know how we Yampolskys are. We're tough people." She asked me not to tell Marty. I wasn't intending to.

When I called Marty late Friday, Vilunya answered the phone and asked if I could call later. She said that they had removed the gastric tube and it was making him nauseous. Before I could hang up I heard his voice in the background asking for the phone. "Hi, boichik," he said, in a strained voice. We spoke for a minute, no more. He was feeling a wave of nausea. Vilunya reported that everything else was going well. They had removed the I.V. in his neck; used to give him blood quickly during surgery should he have needed it. I told Vilunya we would call the next morning so that Arline could speak to Marty also. All was well. I went to sleep that night apprehensive, but believing in the doctor's forecast.

Marty's phone did not answer. Arline and I speculated that he was either in the bathroom (a harbinger of recovery), walking through the corridors or having some tests done. Shortly thereafter Vilunya called. She abruptly told Arline to get me on the line so she would not have to repeat herself. It was a Friday.

She was shaken, her voice quavering. "Marty's been taken to Intensive Care. His hematocrit fell to 18, (dangerously low), and they wanted to determine the cause of the drop and to give him some blood."

"Where are you now?"

"I'm calling from Rita and Randy's house. They live in Branford, 12 or 13 miles from New Haven. I had been trying for an hour to reach Marty before I went to visit him and finally called the nurses' station." She said that the cause of the fallen hematocrit could only be either that he was bleeding internally (deemed unlikely by the surgeon because of the absence of bleeding the days before) or the leukemia. Vilunya said she would call us from the hospital as soon as she learned something.

She called an hour or so later to tell us that the surgeon was going to see him and withdraw some fluid from his belly to see if there was any blood in it. Rappeport, who was advised of this turn of events, said that he doubted the 18 reading. Vilunya was somewhat recovered by this time, a little steadier. She said she'd let us know as soon as she did what was going to happen next. We waited for a couple of hours or more, Arline and I vacantly playing chess. I finally left the house to do an errand and go to my office to finish up a few things. In the back of my mind, although Arline actually voiced it, was the thought that I might have to accelerate my trip and I didn't want to have to stop on the way to the airport if I had forgotten anything. Why was I not going to the airport now? Why was I waiting until my scheduled flight time on Monday? I could save a day and a half if I left now. It would probably double or triple the price of the ticket if I left now instead of Monday. The price of the goddamned ticket! What the hell was I thinking of? What if Marty were to die between now and Monday? How would I feel then? What the hell's the difference, I told myself, if Marty died before I left or if he died while I was traveling to New Haven or sitting in a waiting room outside his room? If Marty dies, the Angel of Death will cover me with the same black wing he covers Marty, creating a blackness that admits no light, no voice, no connection with the world just departed.

When I checked in with Arline after arriving at the office, she told me that Vilunya had called and told her that Marty was in surgery. I tried to hide my tears from Arline. "Poor Marty," I said.

My first image was of Marty having to undergo everything all over again; all the anticipatory fear and anxiety and then the terrible physical assault. As events unfolded it seemed that, although it was different from the first surgery, it was as bad as I had imagined. Marty had become Dad, unconscious, in a "paralyzed" state, entubated, like Dad just before he died -- no longer competent, not able to direct events or alter them in any way, not even to beg for a change.

In the summer of 1982 I had gone on a ten day horseback trip through a wilderness area in Wyoming with my son, Jonathan, still a graduate student in Economics. When we returned to the lodge outside Cody, there was a call from Phil who told me that Dad had suffered a deep cortex stroke while on a bus tour through the Canadian Rockies with Mom and Arline and her parents. Arline had called Marty, who met her in Jasper and, together with Mom and a Canadian nurse, had escorted Dad back to a hospital in Los Angeles. He had almost died on the plane and was not expected to last long. That was early August. He lived till mid-October.

The stroke left him unable to speak, swallow, self-locomote or move his bowels. He had pneumonia and other problems that his doctors, with downcast eyes and grave tones suitable to the tragic circumstances, assured us would end his life soon. One doctor, to whom I tried to explain something about Dad's will and motivations, interrupted me and abruptly demanded that I not use the present tense when referring to him. "Don't say your father is, he was! He's finished. He'll never recover." Although his comments were like a glove in the face, after some minutes I found myself appreciating the forthrightness of the young, tall, rangy, doctor. They were all wrong, however. His pneumonia cleared up as did his other problems. What was left was a healthy 86 year old man whose only problem was that he had to live as a helpless infant.

Our dad, Moish, with barrel chest and powerful arms and shoulders and standing at five foot six, who I had seen stretch a man six or seven inches taller than he, holding him by the throat while he stuttered the vilest insults he could think of. Our dad, to whom no horse was too wild to ride or to whom no nut, no matter how old or frozen, could resist the power he put behind the wrench he wielded, who the year before, visiting in Phoenix, chased a jackrabbit we had startled while walking in the desert, leapt washes and charged through greasewood, finally stopping, worn out, with a look of savage, joyous satisfaction illuminating him, could not accept staying alive helpless, dependent and without dignity. The problem was in communicating with him.

There he sat, propped up with pillows, one hand and arm lifeless, the other almost so, his body threatening to teeter over, his breathing labored and whistling alongside the feeding tube, his eyes, now focused, now vacant, now pleadingly bewildered. I was positive he didn't want to stay alive this way but couldn't devise a way to communicate with him. One day the night nurse told me she had presented dad with a kind of Ouija board and invented a game with the letters that permitted him, in moments of lucidity, to spell out words and phrases.

As soon as I was able to be alone with him I wrote out an alphabet and asked him to indicate which letter he wanted. Through grunts and eyelash openings and closings denoting negative and affirmative responses we began to communicate. When I was sure that his letter selections were meaningful and not random, I asked him if he wanted to continue to live. I trembled at the impertinence of the question. I wished that he would have slapped me across the room and roared his disapproval of the liberty I had taken. Instead he spelled NO. I repeated the question. He answered the same. I asked him if he wanted to die. He spelled YES. I repeated it and he answered the same. There was no mistaking his wish. I took his hands in mine, pressing them against my cheek, his strong, work-scarred hands, and told him, through my tears, that I loved him and that I would help him to die. His eyes glinted with appreciation, with something that approached gratitude. Not gratitude for my help, but for the realization that he still had some power left to command his environment. I left his room, brushing past his nurse to find a quiet place in the visitor's waiting room to compose myself and think about how to fulfill my promise.

To verify that Dad had truly asked to die and that I had understood his request accurately I asked Phil and Marty to conduct their own interview with him. They did and reached the same conclusion. Without having a precise plan but with the notion that I was seeking advice, I sought out the doctor who had given me the brutal reminder that Dad could never recover and began telling him of Dad's wish. Before I could finish, but when my meaning was becoming clear, he broke loose from our huddle and ran down the hospital corridor shouting over his shoulder, "Get away from me. Don't ever come near me. Don't talk to me. Stay away from me. Never mention that again."

I can't remember many lower moments. I had promised something that I might not be able to deliver; something of the greatest consequence to my father's life. I could barely concentrate on the daily round. When I would catch Dad's eyes following me across the room I imagined a hard, accusatory beam focused on me. I was a patricide, an incompetent one to boot. My thoughts became wild. If I couldn't enlist the help of the doctors I would have to do it myself. I could get poison and administer it to him. I could tell him what I was doing and give him a chance to back out. Where would I get the poison? I didn't know. I could smother him with a pillow. Could I? Could I, feeling his powerful body convulsively struggling to draw breath while I snuffed his life out? Even in his debilitated condition was I strong enough to do it?

Ultimately, I discussed the matter with a doctor friend. I spoke in generalities, describing the situation. He asked me specific questions about Dad's condition. What was really on my mind, although I wasn't sure I could utter the words to anyone else, was to ask my friend for a poison I could administer. Before I had to, my friend said, "Tell your father's doctor that he is in pain and he needs a morphine drip." I told him that it wasn't true. To the best of my knowledge he wasn't in pain. Why then, I questioned, should he need a morphine drip? "Tell your father's doctor that he is in pain and he needs a morphine drip," my friend intoned. I offered more objections, more arguments. He repeated his advice, in an affectless voice, with no variation, syllable for syllable, word for word. This went on for several more times until his meaning began to glimmer dimly in my mind. I stopped talking and thanked him.

When I repeated the coded dialogue verbatim to dad's doctor, with no further discussion he gave instructions to remove the feeding tube and installed an I.V. through which they began dripping morphine. They placed him in a supine position and, almost immediately his face assumed an intent, contemplative mien, as if he were thinking of a chess problem. He opened his eyes from time to time during those next five days and sighed deeply, seeming to relax deeper and deeper into his journey. He was leaving us. We knew it and it seemed to each of us at moments during the process, that he knew it too. He would not go punctured by a forest of desiccating wires and tubes, observed by an audience of mocking gauges and dials, struggling in his own waste, ugly and disrespected. He was going gently, his family watching over him, thinking and feeling and sometimes speaking our good-byes, the old Pharaoh being borne respectfully to his sarcophagus. His brow unfurled, his breathing became rhythmic, steady, pronounced. Phil, Marty, Arline, Mom and I watched his breathing progressively slow. We heard the onset of the death rattle, less dramatic but more elongated than I had thought it would be and we were there the moment he stopped breathing. We kissed him goodbye moments after he departed for death. Arline, who loved my father as much as her own, and who had been with him when he was stricken in Canada, softly said, "Thank God," through her tears.

Marty's surgeon, it turned out, had found blood in the "core sample." She took him directly to the operating room and opened him. I found out later that "opening him up" was somewhat easier than the horror I had conjured. After Phil told me that the incision could not have fully closed in the five days since the initial surgery I began to think of it as unzipping.

Then came the word that he left the paralyzed, sedated state of anesthesia. We waited while the machines sustained him. "His signs are steady," said his nurse, meaning his heart (after ventricular tachycardia and a chest-pounding we found about later), lungs, and kidneys (after "difficulties"). Maybe tomorrow they will remove the breathing tube so that he will be able to talk again. Observation for a day in ICU and then back to a room. Wait Marty, hold on, I'm coming. You are not Dad, you're young, you're not really paralyzed. I'll be there soon. When I get there I'll help, I'll give you... what will I give you? A picture of your healthy self, a healing kiss, my tears. I don't know, but it will be good for both of us.

The flight that I was scheduled to take to Boston on Monday was canceled. I immediately blamed myself for being irresolute and not leaving on Saturday, and promised myself a dire punishment if I ever behaved that way again. I was able to board a flight that left just two hours later and called ahead to let Vilunya know of the change of plan. She told me that Dara, a young friend of theirs, was going to New Haven that night and would pick me up and drive me down. What good news that was. It would relieve me of many arrangements: luggage and transport from airport to train and then from train to hospital in New Haven in the middle of the night. When she met my plane Dara immediately told me that Marty was holding his own.

The better than two-and-a half-hour drive was good for me. I knew from the information Dara had given me that I would see Marty alive. The noisy heater in her car comfortingly poured warm air on me, soothing and permitting me, I realized, to unclench my body for the first time in two days. We talked, almost exclusively about Marty and the effect Marty's illness had on Vilunya, Aaron and Leah. Dara had been close with Leah since early adolescence and knew their family well. I had met her several times before. Her comments about them were perceptive, and I thought, discreet. She didn't know me well enough to be more frank, but from what she didn't quite say, I gained the impression that strains were developing within their family.

The undulating countryside flew past. The night was illuminated alternately by the moon and, infrequently, by the garish blast of lights announcing rest stops. Occasional houselights, seen twinkling in the distance through the leafless woods, seductively promised warmth and comfort from the mid-December night cold. When, from time to time, meadow or field opened to the side of the highway, a slash of moon reflecting on the softly lying snow shot through the windshield, and as quickly as those moments appeared they vanished in the wake of our speeding car and we were once again plunged into the wooded dark. My eyes needed a brief time to adjust to the blackness, able only to see the path blazed by the car's headlights. Even when I couldn't see it I knew that there was habitation beyond the range of my vision; farmsteads, villages, clusters of houses, crossroads taverns, proofs of continuous settlement for three hundred years and more. It comforted me to believe that all around were generations of people who had continuously dwelt here, building the country for their use and enjoyment and that of strangers like me who would pass through on highways built by their hands.

I fell into a romanticized revery, lulled by the steady sonority of the engine and tired by the full day of travel. I imagined Marty's doctors: New Englanders, spare of word, brilliant in their approach to his problem, caring in their treatment of him, flawless in the strategy they were employing to cure him. The fantasy was becoming as delicious as I knew it to be unrealistic. Still, it relaxed me to think that Marty was in good hands, recovering even as I was driving to see him. He was alive and I would see him soon.

Piercing the uterine solace of my thoughts was the memory of being greeted by Marty at the airport in Los Angeles and the trip to the hospital to see Dad for the first time after he suffered the stroke. Marty tried to prepare me for how Dad looked. He began with a grave expression, giving me headlines about Dad's loss of various functions. He could see, however, that I could not correctly visualize the situation and, to avoid my being shocked more than was necessary, he mimicked Dad's condition. With wild eyes and spastic movements of his head and arms he let me know that I should not expect to see, perhaps ever again, our Dad. As Marty grimaced, we simultaneously experienced the childhood feelings of guilt and fear when Dad was angry at us and bore down upon us with a rage that he could not suppress. Marty and I tried to maintain respectfully blank demeanors while his face contorted with the effort of attempted speech as he made guttural grunts of the accursed consonants he could not overcome. Our fear was of letting out the laughs we were stifling and facing annihilation at his violent hands. At the crescendo of his rage and hurt feelings he would either banish us or administer a furious, albeit quick, beating. We always knew, however, that we could not avoid hurting his feelings. That was never our intent, but in those highly charged moments, there was never any discussion, only a storm of fury and sullen silence afterward.

Our nervous joking subsided and gave way to questions and answers about the physical arrangements and the doctors' reports. And then we lapsed into a silence, each to prepare to face Dad. I thought then, as now, speedily approaching New Haven in the cold night, about what my reaction would be when I saw him, what it should be, about how those around would react. Should I cry? How much should I cry? Should I restrain my tears? Should I let them flow and even pour more out so that all of us in our little family could express our feelings without restraint, could express our fears, our grief, our helplessness? I tried to prepare.

Intensive Care Unit, or ICU, is always alive with activity because death always hangs in the air. Every movement of the people who work there, every device for monitoring and communication as well as the very physical layout of the unit is designed to fend off death. Each patient is in a tiny cubicle crowded with equipment and machinery close at hand in preparation for the worst. The place throbs with urgency, sometimes frantic, desperate, noisy, brusque: shouts and movements that signify the battle being lost and death winning. Tubes and wires and equipment of every description are arrayed everywhere in a seemingly haphazard fashion.

A visitor has to be announced through an intercom and given permission to enter. The intercom is in a visitor's lounge which usually is full of family members of ICU patients slumping or dozing on the plastic, cigarette-scarred couches and chairs or idly watching television, numb and exhausted in their anxiety.

Marty's room was beyond half a dozen others identical to his. In some, people were lying alone, motionless in their beds, huddled in pain and delirium. An Asian man, standing beside the bed of a woman so tiny her bed looked unoccupied, stared confusedly at the life outside of his lonely waiting place. Other rooms had elaborate metal constructions, suspending shattered limbs in healing positions. One man lay with legs spread apart, his catheterized penis and fiery, swollen scrotum gaping at passerbies.

At the threshold to Marty's room, before I could scan the array of machines that surrounded him, his febrile eyes fixed me with a gleam of recognition and gratitude. He was alive and now he knew that I knew it. Vilunya and Leah were there with him and wordlessly greeted me with their eyes and soft smiles. I approached slowly, delicately, not wanting to disturb any of the tubes and other apparatuses he was connected to. I took his hand. He beckoned for me to come as close to him as possible, to put my face to his. We kissed each other. I rested my face gently against his. He said to me, in a rasping sob, "I'm so glad you're here." As I greeted him with breaking voice the ravenous rat in my stomach began to dematerialize. As that insatiable, malevolent rodent with metal jaws and fangs faded away for the first time in days, I was able to feel something other than fear. I kept my head and face against Marty's for some time, stroking him while he held me feebly, until, at last, I straightened up so that we could look at each other, weakly smiling. I embraced Vilunya and Leah, in turn. I felt a birdlike tremor in each of their bodies, the fluttering anxiety of the past few days.

Marty was alive. Badly damaged. Badly bruised everywhere. Foley catheter in his penis. An intravenous device (IV) in his neck with three lumens. IVs in his hands. Blood pressure device illuminating his finger. Inflatable device on his ankles and calves for circulation assistance. Fanglike marks on his neck where IVs had been removed. Black and blue patches of hematomas on his hands, wrist and arm where they had failed to find the vein for the IV. His hair was wild; his eyes wilder with recent memory of frightening things only he had seen and felt. He looked more like a trauma victim than the recipient of a surgical "insult." But he was alive.

I repeated it to myself, over and over again. Inspecting him to confirm my understanding, I noted the movement of his toes, his hands, his eyelashes. The four of us, Vilunya, Leah, Dara and me stood close and exchanged the smallest of talk. They questioned me about my trip, my family. I questioned them about Marty. I looked at Marty as Vilunya answered. Although Marty couldn't talk because of weakness and pain in his throat caused by the recently removed gastric tube, his expressive eyes gleamed at me with confirmation of Vilunya's answers or a comic indication that she was inaccurate. Even without voice he eagerly joined the discussion. He reached his hand an inch or two toward mine with a smile. I took it. It felt more like a claw. He tried to squeeze my hand but didn't have the strength. Gradually, he drifted toward a sleep that wouldn't last long and our conversation subsided. In between the quiet words and glances we exchanged I surveyed the bewilderingly crowded ICU cubicle.

Marty's bed was really a working slab with infinite adjustment possibilities to permit the medical personnel to manipulate him easily. His comfort was not at issue. He was too exhausted with his struggle to stay alive to be concerned with comfort. The devices surrounding him measure the responses of his vital organs and enclose equipment needed for emergency treatment. All cubicles are open so the medical personnel can see the patients at all times and, as the need often arises, fly into a room and try to keep life going a while longer.

A man with a grotesquely broken leg, hoisted in the air, with metal pins every few inches, called in a weak and pained voice, "Help, help me. Please help me" for perhaps 3 or 4 minutes. Several doctors were standing within 15 or 20 feet of his room. No one made a move to help him. A nurse, an Irish woman with a fresh brogue, was attending Marty at that moment. Vilunya told her that the man was asking for help. Grunting acknowledgment, she finished her task in Marty's room, and some five minutes later, went to the man calling for help, past the chatting doctors and lowered his leg slightly. He stopping crying for help. ICU is set up for survival. It is a place of desperation, a place in which the only counter to pain and madness are the drugs and the sporadic tender ministration of the nursing staff.

The drugs that lessen the physical pain are necessary. Pain interferes with everything; with communication, diagnosis, with healing, with dignity.

But the drugs, the analgesics, the narcotics, also distort the thoughts as they camouflage the pain. Especially the anesthesia for the surgery. Some of them render the patient paralyzed for obvious reasons. Other drugs render one unable to feel pain and yet others make you unconscious and unable to remember the surgery.

Sometimes, as happened to Marty, the senses, hearing and sight, return before the surgery is finished. His mind as well as those senses was functioning, poorly probably, but he was aware of conversations, and most horribly, he heard the surgical team, in their clipped, survivalist, abbreviated exchanges say that they were losing him, that he was dying.

Randy, a surgeon himself, Marty and Vilunya's friend, told us that in very long surgeries, such as heart replacements, it used to be fairly common for the patient to wake up in the middle of the surgery and be fully aware of everything going on around him.

As Marty was beginning recovery in ICU from the second surgery, especially when he was either drifting off to sleep or awakening from a short, fitful nap, his mind was mangled. He couldn't tell, initially, whether he was living one of his nightmares, the awful, frightening imaginings while sedated, or partially so. In those "dreams" he heard around him ("we're losing him"), ("watch the heart monitor, don't take your eyes off of it"). He someone saying how badly he smelled and hearing patients described as assholes. He remembers being thumped on the chest in the operating room when they thought they were losing him. A young resident told Marty later, in my presence, that he thumped him because he was suffering a "fatal arrhythmia."

Marty "remembered" being in a "safe house" in Newbury Street in Boston where he was being tortured. The safe house came from the stories he had heard from people who had suffered during the violence in Central America. He had known people engaged in clandestine activities, both Salvadoran and Sandinista guerrillas, some of whom who later became refugees. He spoke to people whose ill fortune was simply to be in the path of the conflict. Everywhere he traveled in Central America in the eighties he heard tales of murder and torture. I wondered whether, when he was still anaesthetized, he thought himself a captured combatant being tortured.

When he was taken to ICU from surgery on Saturday night he still had the breathing tube in his throat and could not speak at all. He was extremely frightened and anxious from his experience and he desperately wanted someone to stay with him during the night. Because he could not make his wishes known he had to watch everyone desert him. The next night, Sunday, after his breathing tube was removed, he was able to tell Vilunya and she and Leah stayed with him all night. I asked him if wanted me to stay with him Monday night, the night I arrived. He said he did, at least till he fell asleep. I stayed, as did Leah, till 4:00 AM.

I held his hand a lot that night, his skinny, weak hand, punctured and discolored. I watched him while he nodded off a number of times, entering a state that could not rightfully be called sleep. It was shallow and fitful, seldom lasting more than ten minutes. His cheeks would puff up, bellows-like, and then would be sucked into the bony structure of his cadaverous face. During the sleep he would twitch like a kitten whose nervous system is not yet quite formed. I waited until he had received a shot of Morphine and one of Benadryl and faded into something that more resembled a real sleep. I left weary and relieved.

I went to the house of Rita and Randy, friends of Marty and Vilunya's. Randy is chief of surgery at St. Raphael's, a large hospital in New Haven. Randy and Rita had spent part of the year before in Zimbabwe where he had worked, for local wages, as a matter of principle, teaching native doctors surgery.

When Rita heard of Marty's situation and the plan to have both the splenectomy and the marrow transplant in New Haven she invited them to stay with them in Branford. From the first visits to New Haven and through the ordeal of the splenectomy they made their house available to all who came to support Marty. Although we had never met, they welcomed me into their house. They are straightforward, kind and decent people.

Leah and I crept in as noiselessly as we could just before dawn. The cold penetrated my clothes as I negotiated the short distance between the car and the door. The house was a short distance from Long Island Sound and the insistent, icy wind had no mercy on me until I closed the door behind me.

Rita incorporated me into the breakfast bustle the next morning without ceremony. She showed me how things worked. I joined the others completing their toast, coffee and newspaper articles. That was that. It was perfect for me. I didn't realize till that moment how comforting it was to me not to have to negotiate with a hotel reception desk or a coffee shop.

After breakfast, Vilunya, Leah, Dara and I went to the hospital together. Marty was still in ICU. Glad to be surrounded by us, he seemed brighter. His speech was improved. His throat hurt less.

119

We spent the day seeing to his needs, calling a nurse when needed, giving him water, talking to him. Marty was observing us all. I could see how it hard it was for him to balance his great need to be ministered to—everything from rest and silence when he needed it to conversation when he needed that. He asked a lot of questions. He needed to know as much about his environment, about himself, his condition, as possible. He had to be sure that he was still here, still alive, that there was nothing about his state that was being withheld from him.

I was learning the terrain of the ICU. Several of the cubicles changed occupants. Some left because they were well enough to be transferred to rooms that did not require special care, others died. The culture of the ICU revealed itself immediately. On the one side of the glass and curtain partition were the patients, the helpless ones, connected to life only by the machinery they were attached to.

The other side was the domain of the living, of the competent, of the caregivers. That area, between the patient's cubicles and behind the arc of the desks where reports were made and orders written, was the passageway and congregating area for the nurses and technicians and doctors passing through. They were the ones who monitored the machines and decided when help was given and when patients were doing well enough not to need help. They spoke and laughed loudly with each other, not caring who heard them.

Comparing Marty to the other ICU patients permitted me to conclude that he was stable, but only then did I fully realize how close he had come to death. The splenectomy, supposed to be a beneficial step along the way to the bone marrow transplant and hopeful cure, had almost ended everything.

Doctor Rappeport came by in the afternoon. After he spoke to Marty for a little while, his hand resting on Marty's arm, his eyes constantly surveying the monitors, he stepped outside the cubicle to speak to us all. It was a difficult moment. We were assembled just within Marty's vision, just beyond his hearing. Although Marty's room was too small to accommodate us all comfortably, and standing in the hallway was the logical thing to do, it seemed to me that Marty was being needlessly isolated from the rest of us. I was meeting Rappeport for the first time, the doctor in whom our hopes for a cure for Marty rested and could not bring myself to suggest that we move either into the room or further down the hall so I, along with the others stood outside of Marty's room and passively listened to Rappeport hold forth.

Joel Rappeport, a dark, thin man in his early fifties, always seemed to be seeing or considering something not immediately present, beyond the obvious. Whether seated or standing he slouched, his head cocked so that his body looked misaligned, a praying mantis awaiting opportune prey. Although he moved rather slowly, his speech and movement hinted at a nervous trembling energy, successfully being suppressed by the force of his will. I never saw him when he wasn't at least slightly disheveled, his graying, black hair standing at whatever angle and arrangement his last finger combing left it, his tie at various angles to his customarily unbuttoned collar, and either the stains or remnants of the only food I ever saw him consume; doughnuts, salt crackers or coffee. It was also obvious that he was at least partly aware of how he looked, approved of it and did not object to the impression he was creating. If his manner wasn't exactly warm, it was comfortable. Marty and Vilunya felt at ease with him as I did when I grew to know him. Between us we affectionately called him "Rap" or "the Rapman" or "the Rapster". Face to face we called him Doctor or, at his suggestion, Joel.

That day, after a few general comments about Marty, Doctor Rappeport spoke about the transplant unit and, affectionately, about his close colleague, Brian Smith. He launched into a series of crude stand-up comedian jokes about Marty and me—twin jokes and comments. "I thought Marty looked bad till I saw you." I concluded that he was nervous himself and that he was establishing quickly that Marty was his patient, not I. His duty was to care for his patient, not for me. I was in no position to take offense.

For a number of days Marty experienced periodic returns to the terrifying state that he had been in immediately after the surgery and still feeling the effects of anesthesia. He asked me, in a conversational tone, a question about Jacob Solloway, a boy we had both known in the fourth grade. He caught himself after he said it and remarked very matter-of-factly that he had slipped momentarily into the "other world."

Marty told me some time later that he felt, at times, as if he had "dual citizenship," alternating between the daily, mundane land of health and, when in pain and despair, distantly quarantined. No one, neither family nor friends, had the proper visa to visit him when he traveled to those darker regions.

"Have I been acting like a curmudgeon," he asked me without preamble. His eyes shone with expectancy, anticipating an answer.

"Yes, at times," I said, thinking specifically of orders he had barked at Vilunya and Leah.

He made a slight head movement, confirming the accuracy my reply. "You can't know how different your view of me was from my view of you. It's been very hard for me. My throat ached from where the breathing tube was and it hurt like hell when I spoke. Talking, in general, knocked me out. When I needed something I used abbreviated phrases and sentences. They must've seemed like commands." The explanation tired him.

"Don't worry about it, mano. Save your strength to defend yourself for when I start giving you hell." I took his hand in both of mine and we smiled at each other.

Leah and I went in to the hospital, rather late in the morning. We were both tired from the day and night before. I felt cramped and exhausted and slightly disoriented over the complete newness of my environment and assaulted by the ferocity of the cold I was not accustomed to. Marty had been transferred from ICU to a surgical ward that morning. This would be his first day in a semi-private room, proof of the progress of his recovery. He no longer needed the life-supporting machines.

Entering the huge, out-of-scale, atrium lobby one was attacked by a ferocious cacophony of voices. People were broken field running to the gift shop, the coffee shops, administrative offices, asking directions, visiting with patients temporarily liberated from their rooms. I saw the same patient days in a row standing in the middle of the flow of foot traffic, near the entrance, in hospital gown and bathrobe, clutching his IV stand with one hand, smoking a cigarette and sawing the air with the other, screaming a torrent of obscene invective at no one in particular and demanding cigarettes from passersby. The elevators and corridors were clotted with people all day. Phalanxes of earnest young interns and residents and students vied for lane space with maintenance and housekeeping employees, therapists on the go, visitors seeking their sick relatives and the odd patient risking the traffic to relieve the boredom of the ward.

Entering the warm building from the cold made me clammy. To relieve the feeling I peeled open some of the clothing layers I had recently donned. Enthronged in the moving mass I noted, almost clinically, how anxious I was. My respiration was rapid, my pulse pounding in my ear, my hands wet. What do I have to be anxious about I asked myself? Marty was responding well to treatment. He was on the mend. It came to me in that moment that I didn't trust what I saw and had been told. Deep in a cave in my being, where intuition is indistinguishable from fearful, primitive superstition, where bargains (seldom kept) are made with gods, I reckoned it more than possible that terrible news would await as long as I visited in the hospital. I could never rid myself of that apprehension. Every morning as I approached his room I felt that flutter in my chest even if the news of the previous day was good, as if having a cheerful attitude would be hubristic. Calm would return only after I entered Marty's room and saw for myself that he was still there and at least as well as I had left him the day before.

He did indeed look much better than the day before. He was propped high on his pillows, looking alert. He still had the Foley catheter, the inflatable pump around his ankles, the blood pressure monitor on his finger, but the hope was in the air that these devices would fall away quickly as proofs of Marty's recovery. His smiled greeting to us as he turned off the television with a flourish that was almost a brag about his rapid improvement. As the day wore on, though, his spirits and his energy flagged. Movement of any kind was painful and tiring. Healing was exhausting.

I quickly settled into the new environment, beginning at once to learn the new indices of Marty's health, the new daily round. The surgical ward that Marty's room was in was a vastly different place than the ICU. Here, a semblance of normalcy was restored. Food was served at regular, predictable intervals. Medical personnel came to the room and addressed the patient and waited for the patient's response instead of merely reading charts, making deepthroated sounds for no one's ears and looking at the patient over the top of half spectacles. Television sets blared, patients read, wrote letters, walked slowly around the ward, circumnavigating the command center. Within a day or two certain people, seen repetitively, began to become recognizable. This nurse was bright and cooperative, that one dense and surly, never let that doctor try to insert an IV-he'll give you three hematomas and still won't succeed -- get the fat nurse with the wild red hair -- she'll do it right the first time.

Marty's room seemed spacious after the claustrophobic cubicle. There was more clearance around the bed, and between the foot of the bed and the wall, underneath the high perch of the television set, were two chairs, a luxuriant touch compared to ICU. Even the drab, almost unintentional paint attempting to conceal the walls' scars and blemishes and the balls of dust peering out from under the bed seemed tokens of contact with the world outside, not a shore of the Styx that ICU was. The corner of the room contained a small ship's cabin sized closet where visitors could store their heavy clothes. Marty's street clothes hung in the closet, optimistically awaiting his discharge. Every day as I hung up my coat and scarf I looked at his pants, shirt and jacket hanging limply, forlornly waiting return to service, I asked myself how long will it be? I asked for my sake as well as Marty's. I had been there four days and it felt like a month.

Marty's roommate, separated from him by a hanging curtain, was a young drug addict in need of a heart valve replacement. He watched television night and day and kept the nurses enraged by consistently calling for his pain medication before he was scheduled to get it while showing no evidence of being in pain. Members of his large extended family would bring him Italian dishes. He was pleasant enough in the daily small talk we made with each other.

Marty was still very uncomfortable, despite being in a bed that could be adjusted to any configuration. He was discovering new sore spots on his body from the surgery and the handling he had been subjected to. He had no appetite and was intermittently nauseated. Without discussing it, Vilunya, Leah and I campaigned for Marty to eat more than the crumbs he consumed before sending back his tray and to force himself off the bed to stroll through the ward as much as he was able. Marty, in a clear declaration of his sovereignty, swiftly let us know that he would be assuming control of his situation. That didn't stop us from pushing, but it did lead to a tense moment or two. I determined to push until he told me to piss off.

A young resident swooped into the room, the hem of his white frock trailing, swept up the chart at the foot of the bed, glanced at it briefly, theatrically, in a way intended to show competence and speed, and said, "How are you feeling, Martin? I'm Doctor Gilchrist. I'll be examining you from time to time. Have you had a bowel movement yet?" He was in his early thirties, athletic looking, with short reddish blonde hair, a scrubbed, reddish gleam to his skin and a bristling, English officer's mustache, upon which he had lavished great attention.

Marty lifted his head off the pillow slowly, rearranged his body laboriously, as if carefully assembling its parts, his attention focusing on the young resident like a buzzard peering at a live animal soon to be carrion. "What is your first name", Marty asked, dryly.

"Leonard," the young doctor responded, with a trapped look. The rest of us looked out the window or toward the door to ease his embarrassment. "No, Leonard, not yet. I haven't had a bowel movement." The doctor advanced, hastily took Marty's pulse, read his blood pressure and pulled the blanket off his feet to observe the ankle pump. "You probably don't need this any more. I'll send someone to take it away. Everything looks good." Attempting a smile that he hoped would erase his blunder, he returned the blanket to its original position, and trying to be brisk and businesslike, left the room quickly, hastened by our mirth, which, we calculated from the quickness of his step, he had divined correctly, would soon turn audible.

I called Arline. I could hear in her voice how happy she was to have Jonathan with her for the week. She told me that her shoulder was better. The break had certainly healed and the exercises were increasing her mobility. Although she never said it, I knew she was worried that she would be left with a dead arm and shoulder, partially invalided. She had had a "frozen shoulder" several years before, a condition in which adhesions form as a result of a traumatic injury, mechanically barring the free movement of the shoulder. For more than a year her shoulder pained her constantly and showed no sign of improving. In her characteristically determined way she faithfully practiced a series of exercises that broke the adhesions and restored full use of the limb.

"How is Marty?"

"He's out of intensive care, in a double room on a ward. The doctors seem to think he's out of immediate danger."

"The doctors seem to think? What do you think?"

"It's hard for me to have an opinion. He's so beat up right now that it's hard to imagine the state he's in being called an improvement."

"How are his spirits?"

"He varies. Sometimes he's fully engaged, other times he's sullen and withdrawn. He still has a lot of pain and his functions still haven't full returned."

"And Vilunya? How is she holding up? Does she show her feelings?"

"She's obviously very relieved Marty's out of ICU. She bustles around a lot, making a convincing show that she is sure everything is going all right. Every once in a while her face twists into a grimace when she sees Marty in pain. Once or twice she clouded up. But you know Vilunya. She doesn't show much. How's Jonathan doing?"

"He's fine. He's right here. He wants to talk to you. Just a second. Take care of yourself, darling. Give Marty my love."

"Hi, dad," Jonathan pealed brightly. "How is everything going there?"

I gave him an up-to-date account, filling him in on some of the background Arline knew but Jonathan was probably not aware of. He asked detailed questions about his beloved Uncle Mighty, the name Jonathan gave him as he was learning to speak. The adult Jonathan, Jonathan the economist, was interviewing me now, carefully researching Marty's condition. He wanted the facts to lead to a conclusion that logically gave Marty's prognosis, and he wanted that prognosis to be optimistic. His questions were always put gently. I told him of Marty's progression, from the cusp of death after the surgery to his present state. Jonathan exclaimed several times when I told him of low points. I told him the trend was up and we were encouraged.

"How are you making it through all of this?" he said in a husky voice. "Are you holding up okay?"

"I'm doing all right, son. Being here and seeing for myself is a great help to me. Just knowing instead of letting my mind run wild is a comfort to me."

"Dad, I don't know if this is the right time to tell you this and I sure wish it could have been in person. Diane is pregnant. We confirmed it just last week."

"Oh, Jonathan! Of course it's the right time. It would always be the right time for such good news, but especially now. We're all in need of some good news. How is Diane feeling? Is everything okay with her? How are you feeling? Are you both excited? When will the baby come? I'm going to be a Grampa. Can I tell everybody?"

I could feel Jonathan's smiles through the phone at my torrent. "Yes, dad, everything's okay here. Diane is feeling great. The baby is due the end of July. We're both very happy about it. The doctor says everything is going fine. Sure, tell everybody." Arline picked up the extension phone and we roared kisses and hugs between the three of us, Arline and I calling each other Grandma and Grandpa over and over. I walked back to Marty's room slowly, trying to calm my excitement. I was thinking about how to tell them, or whether to tell them, the wonderful news, right now. What concerned me was the terrible contrast. My immediate family just received such joyous news while Marty's was struggling with its terrible crisis. I wanted no hint of a rank to be present.

Vilunya could see the light in my face as I entered the room, and before I could speak, she said, "What?" I told them both the news, reportorially, attempting to contain my excitement. Vilunya's face exploded with a shining smile. She came from around Marty's bed, where she had been sitting quietly and hugged me. "Mazeltov, mazeltov," she said. She did a little dance in place. Marty raised himself from his reclined position, leaned forward vigorously and opened his arms toward me. "Oh Sauly, what wonderful news, what wonderful, happy news." Carefully navigating around the I.V. tree and lines I entered his embrace, leaning over the bed. Vilunya followed and the three of us awkwardly hugged.

After only a few days I was becoming part of the life of the hospital and I hated it. True, my title was guest or visitor or family member and not patient, and for that I was grateful. The hospital was drawing me into it; making me part of its quotidian, endlessly repeating, detailed workings. I didn't want to be a part of it. I didn't want Marty to settle deeply into it. I didn't want Vilunya and Leah to become used to it. I wanted us all to be outside, in the healthy world, the world in which the hospital is regarded as a transient episode. I began to carve niches of time and space for myself, places and moments of escape, to seek refuge from the constant, grinding, waiting for a good result, for the news that Marty's condition was improving and a time for his leaving could be established.

That evidence was slow in coming. For the first several days in the surgical ward he looked only slightly better than he did in ICU. The food didn't interest him and a trip to the bathroom exhausted him. Gradually, his guts started functioning again and that was greeted by us all, rejoicing with bad jokes. I could tell that he was worried, although he didn't give it voice. He was monitoring himself, waiting for the ever-present nausea to vanish, for some spark of vitality to return. He still needed painkillers for the aftereffects of the surgery, which was evidenced by the eighteen inch gash on his abdomen, the pinkish upwelling of the scar held in place by large industrial looking metal staples.

Marty wasn't very interested in conversation. He would tire easily, and when he talked too long he would signal his need to disengage by lowering his voice and by the obvious ebbing of his interest in what was being said. He would either retreat into a silent contemplation, fully awake, or try to sink as comfortably as possible into a nap. Those were the times when my spirits sank. I looked at Marty withdrawing and, in an effort not to dwell on the possibility that he might never get better, my mind flew out of the hospital room but could never alight in a more cheerful venue. I would think about business problems that awaited me in Phoenix or how Arline was doing without me. I wanted to flee but there was no escape while Marty was so sick.

A bright spot of those days was associating with Leah, my niece. Our routine for the few days following Marty's transfer out of ICU was for us to leave the Branford house together in the morning. We tried to time our arrival at the hospital to coincide with the completion of Marty's morning ablutions, usually getting there at mid-morning. We would finish breakfast and drive to the hospital through the slush and disappearing snow under the leaden, threatening sky. Vilunya would join us later. For the time I was to be at the hospital both Leah and Vilunya would take a day or two leave to go to Lexington and Cambridge. They needed the small relief and were confident that necessary matters would be attended to while I was there. Vilunya was Marty's advocate while he was too weak to be his own and even when he was strong enough to fend for himself she remained alert to all that had to be done for him. With a fierce determination she made sure that they didn't forget the myriad medical matters such as the time of a certain procedure to be done, a change in medication or a substituted food item. Although most of them could have been described as housekeeping, their sum, I was convinced, could have been the difference between recovery and death. More than once she or Marty discovered the wrong medication as it was about to be administered.

Leah was in a difficult position. Just twenty-seven, she had left California and a stable relationship with a young man the previous summer to come east and live with her folks to help during the time of the transplant. Everyone thought at that time that the transplant would occur mid-winter. Instead, the splenectomy was happening in mid-winter with no way to predict when the transplant would occur. Leah was willing to temporarily sacrifice her independence out of love and loyalty to her family. Her life was interrupted. Physically separated from her boy friend, unable to seek steady, long term, career enhancing employment, she was needed where she was.

She didn't complain about her choice although it must have worn heavily on her. She was almost always sunny, willing, energetic, her white teeth announcing her ready laugh. Slim and attractive, her olive complexion and long, red-flecked, dark brown hair smartly contrasted with the bleached and tired lumpy majority in New Haven, struggling with a long winter. Everywhere we went young men would crane for a look at her, a tribute Leah accepted with quiet confidence and which made me feel protectively proud. When, on occasion, she felt oppressed by Marty's situation, she would withdraw quietly, without a fuss, and reappear after a short time, refreshed.

I had known Leah since she was born, but this was the first time I was encountering her as a fully formed adult. For those few days, until she went back to Cambridge to help out in her mother's shop, and while Vilunya had taken a day or so off, we were in each others company almost constantly. We talked all the time we were not with Marty, driving, having meals in the cafeteria, strolling in the hospital corridors when Marty was sleeping or having some procedure done. We talked of her life, Leah consistently understating the upheaval her return was causing, of the extended family we both belonged to and above all, of Marty, of the particulars of his case, of his progress, of his future. We trudged the corridors of the hospital together, heavy with worry and doubt about Marty, each ready, however, with logic and persuasion to convince the other that the signs were optimistic. We had dinner together one evening at an upscale Italian restaurant and stopped another evening at a workmen's tavern late at night. Standing at the bar Leah shyly asked me for advice about what kind of drink to order; one that did not make her sound like she was unused to ordering alcohol at bars. We remained standing, drinking our drinks, for perhaps fifteen or twenty minutes, surrounded by beer drinking dart throwers, the heavy, dim air reeking of body odors released from heavy clothing used in outdoor work. Leah enjoyed the brief respite from the taxing day. She was poised and worldly, but above all, of ingratiating disposition, not cloyingly or in any way false, simply a reflection of the sweet young woman she had become.

After several days Marty said he was ready to have a turn around the ward. He had shaved and donned a bathrobe he had brought from home. Together, we set out to circumnavigate the central nurse's station.

"I don't want to overtax myself so when I feel I've had enough I'll go right back to the room." He fixed a crooked, humorless, stare at me.

"All right, tell faithful Chang when you want to go back and he will take you."

"I mean it," said Marty, anxiously. I agreed and off we went, Leah, Marty and I, slowly, taking deliberate steps, breathing rhythmically, as in a Zen walking meditation. Marty held me by the arm, like a debutante holding her father. He was noticeably shorter than I, bowing slightly to minimize the tightness and the pain of his midsection wound. During the walk I fully expected Marty to flash a look of evil irony at me and ask why I wasn't able to walk any faster. I was wrong. He had no taste for irony. He had no strength for humor.

Something drew Marty's attention every step of the way. He focused on a scale, a chrome pipe extending from the wall, a missing floor tile. He was curious in the same way our dad had been, hungering to know how things worked, like a child with no experience in the world. Inventorying everything in his surroundings, he still needed proof of the world he had returned to. He was trying not to wince, in lieu of which, slight syncopations crept into his speech as did certain barely perceptible involuntary muscular spasms. He was starting to sweat. Pain and fatigue were overcoming him and we were barely half way around the circle. Marty paused at the beginning of the low counter bordering the nurse's station and leaned against it, one hand still entwined in my arm but now gripping it as tightly as he could, like a bird holding on to a perch, and the other holding the counter for support. He smiled weakly at me, not quite ready to capitulate, not quite sure if he could make it.

"Shall I get a chair?"

"Nah. Just give me a minute to rest."

Marty surveyed the frantic activity in the work station before him and seemed to draw strength from the exertions of the people behind the counter. Telephones were ringing without cease, residents and interns were trying to learn about specific patients by leafing through files and notes, nurses were carrying small medication trays, moving quickly, their rubber-soled shoes squeaking authoritatively on the polished floor. A middle-aged, black nurse, who had attended Marty, seated at a counter in the middle of the station, made eye contact with him and flashed him a smile of encouragement and approval. He acknowledged the contact with a nod of his head and straightened slightly. Food servers were slowly pushing their carts through the traffic to the appointed rooms, the odor of hot generic food wafting in their wake.

After a few minutes of resting and observing, Marty signaled with a hitching motion, that he was ready to resume, and at a slightly invigorated pace, walked back to his room where, without discussion, he slowly mounted his bed and fell heavily asleep. A note was waiting for me in the room from the social worker who was asked to contact me by the Bone Marrow Transplant Unit.

Marylou, the social worker, in her early thirties, greeted me in her tiny office with a firm handshake. She was small and dainty and dressed like she was on her way to a high tea. Her pretty face was almost always illuminated by a smile of good news. Her skin was good and her large, clear eyes, perky nose and girlish mouth were framed by a soft, large curled hairdo the color of dark honey. Her eyes would dim when difficult subjects were discussed.

Marylou, the manicured, we labeled her. She would tell me what support services she was able to offer me or to suggest I seek.

The wall in front of her desk was full of photographs, largely of children, who had been transplant recipients. Most were bald or with a slight fuzz, all with expressions that were supposed to be smiles. They were instead either the dazed look of a child who tries dutifully, without understanding, to execute the orders given, or a painted, smiling grimace from the child who knows what is expected of him before the order comes, or the pained, pathetic look of the hurt child. All the children shown, through their variety of expressions, seemed to be begging the adults for mercy, for alleviation of pain.

The sight of the children's gallery upset me. It was one thing to deal with images of adult leukemia patients risking their lives in a bone marrow transplant to try for a cure, or at least a prolongation of life. If it failed it usually meant that a life would not have been lived to its full span. But for the children who stared at me from the imprisonment of their suffering, an unsuccessful transplant would mean that they would die before they had lived, before they had known what it was to live.

"How many of these kids survived?"

"Plenty, most of them, practically all of them." The question unnerved her. "About ninety something percent."

"How about the ones not pictured on the wall?"

"I don't keep track of them that way. I couldn't say precisely."

Marylou, recovering quickly, was fascinated that Marty and I were twins involved in a Bone Marrow Transplant, a BMT. She had never experienced both twin donor and recipient in the several years she had worked at the hospital. I was getting the impression that she believed that the fact of our twindom placed certain psychological burdens upon me that she would help me to address. Her remarks were larded with references to counseling, therapy and undefined professional psychological assistance. She told me of a friend who had written a masters thesis about thirty-five-year-old twins. When I expressed some polite interest in it she was vague about how to obtain a copy. She dwelt too long and urged too much on the subject of counseling. Her approach began to annoy me. I wanted information about two subjects; lodging during the month I would be in New Haven for the transplant and a tour of the BMT unit. Marylou wanted to delve into the mysteries of twins. She wanted me to open up, to reveal myself. I finally told her that I didn't feel the need at the moment for psychological counseling, but if and when I did I would be sure to let her know. She noted the finality in my tone of voice and said she would arrange a tour of the BMT unit as soon as she could.

I left her office feeling agitated. It was not just the pictures of the leukemia-suffering children. Making an appointment to visit the BMT unit extinguished any flickering doubt there may have existed that Marty was either to have the transplant or die. All the other evidence; the conversations with Marty and Vilunya over the past year or more, the reading I had done, the evidence of looking at Marty, the splenectomy itself which almost killed him, had somehow not completely silenced the tiny buzz of hope I still harbored. The formal recognition of a minion of a great hospital with its huge buildings and assortment of the latest machinery for diagnosis and healing, for computerized billing, for gaining public recognition and the respect that accompanied it, that a Bone Marrow Transplant was to be performed on my brother Marty, convinced me in both my mind and my heart. Its very name, Yale Medical Center, had the majestic ring to it that left no doubt of the authenticity of its voice or the correctness of its pronouncement.

I walked aimlessly through the corridors, unwilling to return to Marty's room just yet for fear that my looks would betray my mood. If Marty survives the aftereffects of the splenectomy, if no complications (ones we haven't even imagined) arise to kill him, if he recovers his strength sufficiently to be submitted to chemotherapy to reduce the tumor burden as a conditioning for the BMT, if the chemotherapy has the desired effect, if the chemotherapy or an opportunistic infection doesn't kill him, and if I'm still alive and healthy enough to be his donor, then, probably within the next year I'll be back in this hospital. What will happen during that time? What will Marty's life be like? Or mine?

How will he, or I, be able to concentrate on the balance of daily life while waiting for the transplant?

Marty would have had a taste of death after the hospital stay. I pictured him back in Lexington, alone, the bleakness of the remaining winter forbidding him access to the outdoors, confronting his weakness and pain, facing an uncertain outcome, but with the certainty of more suffering and more pain. Doubtful of his ability to tolerate the pain and guilty over the torment he would be visiting upon those around him, he would opt not to continue. Not by slamming the newspaper down on the table like our dad would have done, with an " ah for crissakes" that sounded like an iron gate clanging shut and signaling a violent episode, but by simply becoming disengaged, losing interest, saying nothing to anyone, not even me, just slipping away. Or, if he didn't go in that direction, would he be able to think clearly enough to arrive at the right decisions?

During that time I would be conducting my business, which was entering a dangerous time for me, threatening to gut the comfortable retirement I thought my work had made possible. Could I carry on my business with the concentration it required? Would Arline's shoulder heal completely? What of the rest of life; of a grandchild as yet unborn, of the new president, not as yet inaugurated, of books to read, of the basketball playoffs, of growing tomatoes, of traveling, vacationing, playing, enjoying. Could I do those things without being paralyzed by the thought of Marty's pain-ridden body? Would there be a tinge of guilt?

My stomach ached. I felt overwhelmed by the bleak situations I had posited and rapidly, as if from one movie frame to the next, images of a frightening, recurring childhood nightmare replaced the semi-rational thoughts I had been grappling with.

Sabu, in the "Thief of Baghdad," was caught in a giant spider web in what looked like a huge well or a deep, vertical mine shaft. In that dank and fearful place a spider, twice his size, was advancing toward him, its red eyes malevolently gleaming, its powerful beak opening and closing, foretelling the horrible fate soon to befall him. Suddenly, a huge sword comes into Sabu's possession. With it he cuts the strands of the web between him and the spider. At the severing of the last strand, immediately before the spider's hairy leg touches Sabu, the spider falls, slowly, silently, toward the bottom of the almost bottomless pit, to its death. Instead of a fadeout and ending, I am now in the web, glued too securely to move. I have no sword and I will not be able to obtain one. The spider advances on me with sadistic deliberation. Foul, hot odors emanate from its mouth and it touches me probingly with its hairy lance of a leg just before the horror shatters the replay and returns me to the present.

I shudder at these thoughts and consciously struggle to accommodate to the present, finding myself amidst the thrum of activity in the corridor; the sound of wheels and footfalls, the metallic blare of the intercom and the obligato of voices. All around me are the people who make the hospital function. They outnumber the medical staff, although they don't cure anybody. They are the orderlies, the gurney pushers, the maintenance men, the nurse's helpers. Almost all black, they push the carts laden with linens, infected materials, food, patients on their way to procedures. And they clean, removing the ordure of sickness, the deficiency, the unworthiness of ill health and replace it with the competence of starched, brittly clean sheets and the salutary odors, chemically derived, of healthful purity, of nature, free of disease. They dust and they mop and they make beds. When they see each other in passing, each with his own moving burden, they extend greetings with a punctuationless stream of sound, long banners of sounds and smiles floating toward the direction of the listener; the abbreviated talk of the ghetto whose words and sounds are shaped into meaning with well understood gestures. The word languages are Haitian Creole, Caribbean Spanish, but mostly it is the language of the inner city streets, its original southern softness destroyed by the cold, hard life in the northeast.

I drifted along for a time in the current of hospital workers, until I found a small waiting room, one of my spots of refuge. It was empty and I settled gratefully into one of the plastic-covered chairs to make a plan for the rest of my stay. It came to me quickly that no plan was possible. Everything depended on Marty's body healing. That realization gave me a certain comfort, freeing me from further thinking. My head sunk chestward and in moments I was asleep.

Audrey, the head of the nursing staff of the Bone Marrow Transplant unit was expecting me. She agreed to give me a tour of the facility on very short notice, postponing a previous commitment without complaint, but giving me to understand by her manner that there could be no dawdling, just a brisk survey. Without wasting words, she showed me everything, answered all my questions and, waiting a short time to see if I had any follow-up questions, she departed for her appointment. It took a total of about twenty minutes and was entirely satisfying. If the rest of the BMT nursing staff was as skilled as Audrey, I thought, Marty would be in good hands indeed.

There were four Laminar Flow rooms in the unit, lined up next to each other. Between the rooms and the corridor that paralleled them were working areas that ran the length of the unit. On the other side of the corridor was the nurse's station and beyond that, rooms for meetings, supplies and repetitive laboratory functions. There was only one public entrance to the unit so that if someone accidentally strayed into it he was easily seen and quickly asked to leave. A sterile environment was sought for the patient and as clean an atmosphere as possible outside the patient's area.

The rooms were identical; approximately 12' x 10' in size with windows almost the length of the outside wall. One of the walls was a bank of industrial air filters from floor to ceiling. Air from the outside of the room was forced through these filters, trapping solid particles as small as one micron. The fourth wall was made of a completely transparent heavy plastic sheet installed on top of a three foot high solid partition that ran to the door opening. The huge volume of air being pushed through the room escaped through the doorless opening. The rush of air prevented everything but large solid objects from entering the room. No one, not the nurses, not family members, not even Dr. Rappeport, was permitted to enter the room without scrubbing thoroughly and donning a surgical gown and face mask. The patient's bed was immediately inside the plastic wall which had precision openings in it to admit tubes connected to IVs supplying the patient needed medications. In addition, the plastic was penetrated by several arm openings, with built in gloves so that nurses could minister to patients without entering the room and without breaking sterility.

I left the BMT unit with an optimistic feeling. The obvious competence of the nursing staff, the superior medical technology and my perfectly matched marrow, I was beginning to conclude, would stand Marty in good stead for the transplant. As I entered Marty's room I knew, by the black look on his face, that something was wrong.

"Hi, Saul, where've you been?"

"I had a tour through the Bone Marrow Transplant unit. A nurse named Audrey showed me around. It was very impressive. Then I took a stroll around to stretch my legs. How're you doing?"

"Aaah, I don't know. Not so great," he said, screwing his face up into a grimace that let me know something was bothering him, but not volunteering what.

"What's wrong? Are you feeling bad?"

Almost embarrassed to continue, but needing to say something, he said, "It's nothing specific, that is, nothing much feels very different. I'm very weak and afraid."

"Of what?"

"I'm afraid that the same thing that happened last week is going to happen again. That they'll open me up again because they suspect more bleeding and I'll have to recover all over again from another surgery. I don't know if I have the strength."

"Look, Marty, just days ago you had two major surgeries within two days of each other and you're just four days out of ICU. Your body has

135

taken a terrible beating. You've had your guts rearranged, you've lost a ton of blood, you've got what looks like a battlefield wound. Let your body rest a little, restore itself. You haven't been told of any bad signs by the doctors, have you?"

"No." He looked at me questioningly, not sure of whether he wanted to accept my argument, but liking the thread. We were about eye level with each other, he propped up in bed, me standing close to him. He had questions in mind he wanted answered. Specific questions about how soon it could be before he felt better or symptoms he should look for that would indicate something going wrong. He knew I didn't know the answers and I believe he suspected that neither did the doctors. He was content for the moment to listen and draw encouragement from my words. It was an invitation to continue.

I took his hand, gently, careful not to squeeze the hematoma that covered most of the back of it. "Listen, man, you're a fucking horse. After what you've been through, you've made a remarkable recovery. Only two days in ICU, walking around already, of course you're tired. You're made of iron, Marty, but you still need rest. You look better every day since you left ICU. Everybody says so. Just relax a little and get rest. Don't be in a rush. Things are getting better. You'll be out of here before you know it. Your boy is coming in from school tomorrow to see you. The days will get better."

The thought of seeing Aaron soon, something which he had momentarily forgotten, brightened him. "Do you think he'll be able to make it here, with all the flooding I've been hearing about?"

"You know Aaron. He's a resourceful devil. He'll figure it out."

Marty smiled at me. His face was a little sunnier, and the duration of the smile communicated his thanks for the peptalk.

Aaron was coming from his college in upstate New York. His time of arrival was uncertain because of the unseasonable floods. The headlines were full of stories of stranded travelers. Aaron had to take the train to New York City and change for the one to New Haven. Aaron arrived late in the afternoon, joining Vilunya and Leah, who were in the room. Their entire nuclear family was present and I left to afford them a private reunion. An hour later, when I returned, I could see that the mood had changed for the worse.

Aaron was in his second year at college, taking courses in art and sculpture and photography. Since mid-adolescence he had had a contentious relationship with his parents, seeming to prefer argument to cooperation.

He spent a year after high school working at various menial jobs, an experience which everyone calculated was beneficial—teaching him that the world set limits on certain behavior. He worked with tough men on construction jobs and seemed to get along well. So far in college he was successful. He had an active social life, did well in his studies, sang in a student rock band. He was interested in art and showed more discipline in its pursuit than he had ever shown in anything else before. Photography interested him the most, although sculpture fascinated him at the moment.

But this day Aaron was the artist, a role he was playing that looked as if it was lifted bodily out of a bad movie. He was dressed raggedly, deliberately unkempt. Distant and surly, he was rude and disrespectful to Vilunya almost immediately. He didn't seem interested in Marty's condition and he answered questions put to him in a curt and abbreviated way. A suffocating cloud of tension was filling the room. A little tortured conversation was attempted, without success. Leah looked like she wanted to flee. Vilunya's face was pinched and dark. Marty was sitting upright in his bed, stern looking and highly alert, as if ready to spring into combat.

During one of the long silences, Aaron dramatically rolled his pant leg up to his knee and stared intently at what looked like several pimples on his lower leg. He touched them gingerly and winced with pain. He looked around the room, expectantly, inviting some question about his leg. None came. I was standing closest to him and he said to me, in a martyred tone, "burns I got welding. Molten chips burned right into my flesh." He had tried to put a look of agony on his face. He was pleading for someone in the room to discuss his pain, the suffering he had gone through for his art.

Nobody was interested in his complaint. He was sitting a few feet from his father whose survival was still not a certainty. It was the wrong venue to expect sympathy. The more he was ignored, the angrier he became and the more he demonstrated outrageous and childish behavior. I left the room. When I returned some twenty minutes later he was lying in a semi fetal ball on the floor, half his body underneath the bed. Marty asked him what he was doing. Aaron responded unintelligibly and Marty, angrily told him either to behave himself or get out. A few minutes later Aaron left with Vilunya.

Aaron left the next day to return to school. Before he did he and Marty and Vilunya and Leah made attempts to patch things up with softer words. While not successful, the attempt expressed everyone's wish that this not occur again. When I wished him a better visit with Aaron over the holidays Marty said he didn't have the strength to go through scenes like this.

It was Saturday and I was due to leave the next day. I put my reservation up to Monday, hoping the extra days would see the change in Marty that would permit him to go home. My greatest wish was to drive Marty home and see him safely in his bed before I left. I didn't want to carry the impression of him in his hospital room, sick, hurt and depressed.

Marty developed a slight fever that the doctors suspected might be pneumonia. They took cultures from the IV in his neck to see if they could identify the infectious agent.

One of the times I entered the room he and Vilunya were having a grinding, low-voiced conversation. They both had tears glistening in their eyes. Marty asked me to leave the room for a while. When I came back the atmosphere had changed to a cool normalcy. I put my reservation up to Wednesday.

I returned to the house in Branford late that night, tired and dispirited. Randy was still awake, watching the last newscast of the day. When he saw the look on my face he invited me to have a drink and a talk. I accepted both hungrily. Randy is a straightforward person, the way a surgeon is supposed to be.

"I'm worried. They can't seem to identify his infection, much less get rid of it. The fever is still there and Dr. Ward won't release him till he's afebrile for 24 hours. I'm afraid he's slipping, that his body can't take any more.

"Marty will get rid of this infection. He has the strength and the will to recuperate from the splenectomy." Randy drained his glass and covered the reduced ice cubes with scotch. I wanted to ask him about the future, but I had the feeling that he was framing the words he would soon give me. I waited.

"Marty's problems are severe, but they are by no means unique in my experience." His voice was warm and measured. He spoke slowly, part new friend and part seasoned doctor giving advice to a frightened patient. "His real hope lies in the bone marrow transplant. But between now and the time of the transplant you should expect that he will have infections and probably hospitalizations."

"Randy, what do you think his chances are?"

"I think they're good," he replied quickly. As almost an afterthought he said, "First, I believe that he is strong enough to make it to the transplant.

With your marrow freeing him from the possibility of graft versus host disease I think it has every chance to be successful."

Randy's words comforted me. I was buoyed by his confidence in Marty's ability to survive until the transplant. He hadn't told me anything I didn't know and, although his speculations were more informed than mine, he couldn't be sure of the outcome. And yet his words had a powerful effect on me. He knew they would. His timing was perfect and, I am convinced his words were delivered from his heart no less than from his knowledge of medicine.

Tuesday was grim. The black sky drew the light out of the day. Patches of ice were found in seemingly random spots. Although I was concerned about skidding I was having difficulty concentrating on driving. People everywhere were speculating about what the weather would be like the next few days. I didn't care. I had had enough of the bitter cold outside and the overly humid, fart-scented air inside.

I asked Marty how he felt about my leaving the next day. He said he wanted me to stay forever. We both teared up. He explained immediately that he knew I had responsibilities and he didn't want to burden me.

Marty wanted me to stay. He needed me, among others, to help him recover, to keep him company, to minister to him. He and I knew it would help him if I stayed, but it would not be the difference between survival and death.

Our thoughts mirrored each other's exactly. Each of those thoughts, if voiced, would have had a slight rising tone at its end, not exactly forming a question, but, revealing the slightest crack in the surety of the statement. I would, of course, have stayed if Marty's condition required it. *Saul will stay if I seriously ask him to. Marty will understand that I have responsibilities I must return to. He knows I'm not ratting out by leaving. How long can I stay? I know that Saul's leaving means that he thinks I'm recovering. If he didn't he'd stay till he was sure. If I even hint in seriousness that I want him to stay, he'll leave with a sick, guilty, feeling. If I delve any further into Marty's feelings about my leaving he'll become emotional and I'll be left with either having to stay or callously leaving. Everything will change if my/Marty's condition changes.*

After confirming that I could get a flight from Boston at 5:00 P.M. Friday, I called Arline and asked her, in effect, for permission to stay a little longer. I was nervous and a little guilty about staying away so long while she was recovering from her broken shoulder. Jonathan, who had been with Arline for a week, had to return to Cincinnati and his wife, Diane, where, together, they could dream of their baby to come. As I was explaining the situation to her, Arline said to me, almost abruptly, "Your brother needs you and you need to be there with him." When I told Marty of the extension of my stay the news cheered us both up.

Marty's fever was reducing. The surgeon told us he could be released the next day. Vilunya was returning from Boston and Marty brightened momentarily at the thought, although he was still sluggish and withdrawn. He seemed to be discouraged. We didn't discuss it. My guess was that he was frightened about having an emergency after leaving the hospital.

Sitting silently in his room, I reading and Marty in a half doze, we heard live music coming from the ward. It seemed to be Caribbean music, accompanying several less than accomplished voices singing in Spanish. Marty bolted upright in his bed and asked me to find out what it was. Out in the hall was a group of middle-aged carolers, evangelicals from their behavior and dress, sturdy, shabby and somber. They seemed to be playing traditional Christmas carols to cheer up the patients, but in rhythms of sundrenched lands, accented by a *raspa* and *claves*. Of the five or six performers several were singing. About half were black, the others from white to mestizo. The lead singer was a heavy, dark, older woman. In her rendition of Good King Wenceslaus she danced in place, swaying her hips, executing delicate steps and twirling around completely from time to time. The words may have had religious themes but the music and movements were sensuous and decidedly worldly.

As I entered Marty's room to report to him I met him hurrying to leave the room, tightening the belt on his bathrobe and securing his slippers. His face was aglow with happy expectation. I had not seen him move so fast since I arrived at the hospital. We stood in the front of perhaps ten assembled patients some fifteen feet from the performers. Marty beamed. I could feel his body come alive. He was shuffling rhythmically to the music. The piece ended. The short woman singer noticed him and gave him a broad smiling greeting, part maternal and part flirtatious.

The band began a new song. It took them several bars to coordinate their timing and when they had, the woman's voice, hoarse and brittle, burst forth to lead them. Her eyes went from one patient to the next, her voice full of happiness, as if trying to force into her audience her memories of her island, a warm sand beach under a brilliant sky, a time of carelessness, of health taken for granted.

"Dame la mano, paloma, para subir a tu nido." (Give me your hand, my dove, so I can rise to your nest). No Christmas carol this one. The selection animated the whole band. The lead singer's hips were moving without restraint, her feet executing precise, intricate steps, her arms raised from her sides, the pendulous, fleshy hangings following the balletic movements of her hands. She fastened on Marty, her arms extended toward him, her fingers beckoning him. Without coaxing, Marty shuffled across the divide between them, executing a syncopated step along the way, his hands and arms moving both to give him balance and to augment the rhythm. They joined without a word, to the murmured approval of the onlookers. The instrumentalists beamed and formed a semicircle to envelop the dancers with song. Marty had to bend toward the woman to avoid looking over her head. With her face upturned to his she sang to him. They danced for perhaps two minutes. I could see Marty's mouth forming the sounds of the words to the song, tears shining in his eyes. *"Dame la mano, paloma, para subir a tu nido."*

The music ended as exhaustion forced the dancing to subside. They embraced, but before they parted the woman blessed him and wished him well in Spanish. Marty thanked her and trembled slightly from the physical exertion. I made a move toward him, thinking he might fall. He waved me off and walked back to his room, where he climbed heavily into bed. He was too saturated with the moment to speak. We remained in silence till he fell asleep.

Later that day Marty and I strolled around the ward. Although our pace was somewhat retarded because Marty was again connected to his IV tree, he was livelier than he had been in some days. Vilunya was on her way to see him and the music and dancing of this morning had left him with an optimistic glow. We passed an elderly woman, bulldog-faced, solidly built, with a sour expression, dragging her IV tree as she trudged slowly along. As she passed us she looked at Marty, and through a pained smile, said to him, "I seen yez out dere dancin dis mornin. It's what we all need. A few laughs. Y'done good. Good luck t'ya." She sounded as if she knew that the few laughs we all need would permanently elude her, those laughs that I imagined her enjoying in a wooden barroom with peeling paint in a New England mill town where the whiskey laughter inside held the harsh cold outside at bay.

Marty finally seemed to be mending. At least everyone, including him, believed that there was little chance of his condition deteriorating. His temperature was close to normal. And, if the infection was of unknown cause, so what? As long as it was gone. Everyone was ready to get away from the accursed hospital.

Vilunya cooked dinner that night at Randy and Rita's and I arrived in time to join them all for the first time since I arrived. We had wine, and conversation that did not pertain exclusively to Marty, and I laughed without guilt over enjoying something denied to Marty. I felt cheered and confident.

Marty moved very slowly making preparations to leave the hospital. He studied and oversaw every step with gravity, until every arrangement had been made except the actual discharge order: his clothes were packed, his dressings inspected and properly secured, his drug prescriptions in hand, all his questions about every facet of the journey home answered. He was sitting on the chair at the foot of his bed, fully dressed except for his outside heavy coat. Much thinner now than before the surgery, his clothes hung shapelessly from his body. He was sitting tensely, like a guest unsure of his welcome, staring at the unmade bed he had lain in for almost two weeks. Fearfully ambivalent, he spoke very little.

At home he would determine when he would arise in the morning, whether he would lay in bed listening to the radio while he looked out the French door in his bedroom, past the small deck at the fruit trees covered in snow. He would wear his best bathrobe, not the one he brought to the hospital, or he would wear whatever he felt like. His toilet, his telephone, his indoor hibiscus plant in his kitchen. How good that will feel, how much that will promote recovery. Unless, unless. Unless the sharp, but intermittent, pain in his gut that he couldn't even define well enough to describe to the doctors were to turn into a serious complaint. Or unless he developed a genuine pneumonia or a mysterious infection. Or, worst of all, unless the bleeding in his stomach started again. And if it happened at home, could they get him to a hospital in time?

Vilunya, Marty and I made the journey from the room to the lobby together, accompanied by the orderly pushing the obligatory wheelchair. It was almost two o'clock. Each of us expressed the emotional brittleness of the moment differently. Marty was gravely silent. I was quiet, in a state of excited alertness, determined to think of every detail of the trip until Marty would be safe in his own bed. Vilunya was volubly cheerful, ticking items off her list of necessary chores out loud. I went to bring the car from the parking garage after Marty told me exactly how and where to position it. The remainder of the day will be very long, I thought. I ran to the garage, overtaking people along the way. I blew the horn at a driver I thought was moving too slowly in the garage.

The car heater was starting to spread warmth in the car by the time I arrived to pick them up. We helped Marty transfer very carefully from wheelchair to car, elaborately ensuring that the safety belt was securely fastened, a blanket was at hand should he get cold, the seat adjusted for his comfort.

We left New Haven in a light drizzle that couldn't decide between rain and snow, under a pewter sky that made the middle of the afternoon seem like dusk surrendering to night. I was driving with both hands on the wheel, at moderate speed, looking constantly at the mirrors. As we cleared the city traffic and entered the limited access divided highway, Marty said, in a choked voice, "I'm glad to be with both of you going home." Vilunya put her hand on his neck from the back seat and I took his hand, all of us struggling for control. To break the mood Marty turned the radio on. A song came on that Marty identified as Nicaraguan. He said quietly, "I wonder if I'll ever see Nicaragua again?" Vilunya and I assured him, hollowly, that he would.

The drive home took longer than the two and a half hours it was supposed to. The countryside was completely covered with snow. It rained intermittently till we were close to Boston and then a fog descended that reduced everyone's speed to twenty miles an hour and stacked traffic up for miles. Along the way, in western Massachusetts, we stopped at a gas station and convenience market to get coffee. Marty stayed in the car, parked behind the station, looking into the woods while Vilunya and I took turns going inside. When I returned with the coffee Marty was sitting with the door wide open, looking contentedly at the snow-shrouded wood, savoring the ice purified air, unperturbed by the cold, a peaceful expression on his face.

Marty had become an old immigrant, like one of many relatives or friends of our parents or one of the men of our neighborhood when we were boys. Men like our Dad or Uncle Isaac or Sidney Beck or his brother Willie, who we all knew as Velvl, or Mr. Moskowitz, the barber, of whom it was said that his family was so poor and his Polish village so small that he was not even circumcised. Men like these and many others, men of hard lives, who appreciated above all else the absence of war or depression or famine or family tragedy. More than anyone he reminded me at that moment of Uncle Isaac, whom we all loved. I pictured Isaac, in his sixties when we were little, a handyman at a rundown bungalow colony in upstate

New York. His wife Dora, his companion since childhood, had died. Isaac and Dora had had four children, one dying in infancy of pneumonia. The other three, all sons, were our older cousins.

In repose Isaac was flaccid, his pectorals sagging downward to meet his slightly protruding belly, the flesh of his upper arm hanging lifelessly. But when he grasped a hammer or lifted something or braced himself to rise from his chair, a lifetime of hard work asserted its dominion over his body and his muscles, especially his biceps, sprang to full youthful definition. His brown, wrinkled face was illuminated by his thick white hair and drooping mustache, between which his heavy-lidded, oriental eyes shone with proof that his smile was genuine. Isaac showed profound appreciation for the sight of children playing, a breath of fresh air, a drop of whiskey, a peach in season. Like Marty, those old-timers had come from the dead.

What relief and joy there was on arriving home. While I took the bags through the path their neighbor had shoveled through two feet of snow, Vilunya fell, with abandon, to making the house comfortable. She made sure the temperature was adjusted correctly, began preparing food, stacked up the mail, attended to Marty, turned lights on everywhere, checked the list of medications to see whether any of them needed to be taken. Marty sat in a central spot, content to survey the familiar sights from his perch, sights that at times in the past month he must have doubted he would ever see again. Annihilated by fatigue and release of tension, we all went to sleep early.

I woke groggy, disoriented and generally out of sorts. I lay in bed, deferring the moment of separation from the fetal warmth and the frigid embrace of the cold outside, barely held at bay by the window near my bed. I tried to determine why I felt so downcast. Marty was out of the hospital, safe at home and, as I had hoped to do, I had accompanied him on that journey. His survival of the splenectomy was no longer in question. Why then was I not content to leave today with a feeling of satisfaction? I listened to the sounds of awakening in the house. The radio was faintly audible from the kitchen where Vilunya was preparing breakfast. Marty walked quietly past my room and slowly descended the stairs. I was the only one not yet risen from bed. At last, still puzzled by my mood, I arose, showered and shaved, packed, and making a conscious effort to be uplifted and positive, joined them for the final visit of the trip.

Both Marty and Vilunya were glad to be sitting in their own kitchen, around their own table, drinking strong coffee. We talked about Marty's future. He looked gaunt and weak. He had slept fitfully and still had considerable pain in his abdomen, which he alleviated with occasional doses of morphine. Marty was intent on trying light exercise when he was able, to rid himself of the pain. His immediate future would involve chemotherapy when he was strong enough, and if he responded well, to prepare for the bone marrow transplant.

Marty spoke willingly about the future, making time forecasts for each step of the way. He was planning, as his first hematologist had advised him to do many years ago. This time however, his plans did not involve foreign travel for field work or conferences. This time the planning was to stay alive.

Vilunya had gone shopping and Marty and I were sitting in their small, dark, living room. My taxi to the airport would arrive in about an hour and we both found it awkward trying to fill that time with talk. There was nothing we seemed able to say.

My mind was filled with fears and wild fancies. I was Marty's talisman, his magical guide back to the realm of health. As long as I was present and in direct contact with him, he could draw energy and strength from me, enough to compensate for his loss. The donation of fluid, of bone marrow, that would pass from me to him was not enough to save his life. In addition the reserve store of fuel, of life force, that belonged jointly to us would now have to be called upon to see Marty through. How could he recover if I left?

After long silences interrupted by small talk, Marty said, "I'm so glad you came so I could tell you about my suffering." As soon as the words were spoken and heard, the reserve, the holding back, gave way. Unrestrained by the careful attention needed until now to devote to the many tasks leading to the present moment and no longer able to effect the sober demeanor, the long dammed tears rolled down our faces in full flood. We sat and cried. Vilunya walked in at that moment, cheeks happily ablaze with the cold. Her smile faded into a puzzled frown as she looked at the two of us. To answer the question she had not yet asked, I said, "We're just sitting here crying."

The taxi arrived and we hugged and kissed in a mercifully hasty leave-taking. Marty took my hands in his and kissed them. And then I left, trying to think only of the banal conversation I would have with the cab driver to insure against further loss of composure.

WAITING

"Sometimes am I all wound with adders, who with cloven tongues do hiss me into madness." Caliban... *The Tempest*. Shakespeare.

There was no joy in my return to Phoenix. Relief, yes, that Marty was alive when I left him and reasonably expected to remain that way. Also gratitude and the lifting of a weight when I could see for myself the steady progress Arline had made in healing her shoulder. It was plain that she had regained more of the use and mobility in the less than two weeks I had been gone. Parting from Marty left me plagued me with doubts about his future and mine: all the unanswered questions about his present condition and the timing for the BMT and all the steps preparatory to it; the carefully planned steps and the ambushes.

What was he letting himself in for? What was I? I thought for the first time of the part I would play in the BMT. I tried to imagine how they would withdraw my marrow. It sounded painful. I wondered if it would leave me with any permanent impairment. How much warning would I have? Would it mean abandoning an important deal I was in the middle of? Of course there were no answers to these and other questions and fears I had. I resignedly put them away or, more correctly, stored them with the ever increasing pile of unanswered, anxious, thoughts.

Could Marty be saved? The image I carried back of him was of a gaunt prisoner in a concentration camp, peering out between the wires of the fence. He lifts his shirt and reveals an eighteen-inch half moon scar that runs below his rib cage from one side of his body to the other across his yellowed skin. What flesh he has left hangs limply over his revealed bones. His eyes, staring from darkened sockets, ask for help but

146

are resigned to there being none. As I plunge deeper into this depressing hole I picture Marty's increasing suffering with each succeeding procedure. First the agonizing recovery from the splenectomy. Then the torment of the chemotherapy, which works so well it almost kills him. Then the full body radiation preparatory to the BMT. And then the BMT, which doesn't work and he dies.

I wonder if I would be able to live through that sequence. What would it do to me to watch Marty die over the coming year? I would most likely survive it, I tell myself, but the acid I feel in my stomach and the dull ache in my head as I think of it, places that conclusion in some doubt. If something should happen to me, on the other hand, say a rapid episode of illness or a cataclysmic accident, and then oblivion, might it not be better for both of us? No drawn out suffering, just a fast exit. Not so fast, Saul, I tell myself, my interior voice booming so loud a smile forms. Don't be a fucking idiot! You're not going anywhere. Marty is not going to die. He'll get over this surgery, the chemotherapy will be successful and the BMT will work just fine. It will be the triumph of twins that your marrow will insure that Marty lives. If it doesn't, you'll still live. Remember, you and Marty are not Huey and Dewey or Ronald and Donald or the old Welsh farmer twins that Bruce Chatwin writes about in "On the Black Hill," who slept in the same bed till they died in their eighties, or the Australian twin men in their sixties who dropped dead within hours of each other. You are separated, differentiated, two different persons. You'll live. With a pain in your heart, but you'll live.

A day of rest at home with Arline and I thought I would be ready to plunge into my customary, daily life, which, in the time I had been gone, had become distant and unreal to me. The mild Arizona air felt restorative. No bundling up to face the weather, no savage, icy wind tearing at me.

The time I spent in New Haven with Marty was elongated by the minute-by-minute expectation of the worst. When I was outside the hospital I imagined that Marty was gone, just ceased to exist. I would come the next morning and a hospital employee with a doleful expression would tell me in a rehearsed, affectless tone that the management was ever so sorry but Marty, despite their most energetic ministrations, had perished peacefully in the night. No argument on my part, whether quietly reasoned or thunderously roared, could change not only the fact of Marty's demise, but the expression of the teller of the sad news. When I was in the hospital, from time to time an electrical storm of fear would crackle in my stomach, soon accompanied by the almost palpable sound of doctors, nurses, technicians, flying down the hall while the loudspeakers blare, "Code blue, code blue, stat, stat," and give Marty's room number. When that happened I would have to return to Marty's room to look at him, even if he was asleep.

But somehow the intense feelings I had over the uncertainty of his recovery, the savage doubts without rational foundation as to the correctness and efficacy of his treatment, the suffering I experienced just being there hour after hour, became part of a warped equation calculated deep in my emotions, deeper than thought. All of the units of worry, all the small acts I performed on Marty's behalf, all the atoms of fear and anxiety I inhaled and exhaled, would be weighed against the efforts of the dark forces seeking to tear Marty from me. The proof of my victory was that, instead of Charon ferrying a tired and defeated Marty across the river, I had driven him in a Toyota back home to Lexington, Massachusetts. However the gods decide in their juryless court who wins and who loses, they had decided this time in my favor, in our favor. And winning meant surely that not only would Marty be spared but I would draw back from the emotional precipice I teetered on and be restored, for now, to a more stable condition, an alpha state. Things would quiet down, both for Marty, his family and for me. Hah!

I barely noticed the letter from the Circle K Corporation in the two week stack of office mail that awaited me. Circle K was the tenant on a property Arline and I owned; a convenience market with gas pumps. They were about halfway through a fifteen year lease when they filed for bankruptcy, the largest such filing in the history of Arizona. The court gave them the right to decide which of its leases it chose to honor and which it would, in its quaint language, "disaffirm." I was confident that our location was secure because, after a year of bankruptcy they still had not notified us that they were terminating the lease. The short letter I had just read said that they would cancel our lease unless I cut the rent in half.

I have been in the real estate investment business in Arizona since 1960. During that time I have been a broker, earning commissions for selling property for others, a developer of small commercial properties, and since the late seventies, a syndicator of land as well as a buyer and seller of land for my own account. For three or four years during the mid-eighties everything seemed to have come together to produce one large income year after another. I didn't kid myself about why I was doing so well. It was not my genius or negotiating skills or acute analytical abilities, although I was certainly, after twenty-five years of plying it, competent at my trade. The major reason was the tidal wave of enthusiasm that propelled the market, fueled by a seemingly endless supply of cash, provided in large measure, for the first time in my experience, by financial institutions. Sober analysis was discarded, traditional procedures neglected, the most rudimentary investigations overlooked.

I had lived through several cycles before and I knew, with certainty that this one would not last forever. I was cautious. I conservatively selected deals to buy. I didn't hold out for the last bit of profit when it came time to sell. Most importantly, I didn't try to parlay the profits, to let them ride on the next deal, exhausting the cash and assuming more debt. Instead I paid the taxes on the profits, let the cash build up and used a significant portion of it to invest in, what I thought at the time to be secure, income producing properties, leased to good tenants for long enough periods of time to weather the downturn I knew was coming. The income from those properties, Circle K being one of them, was more than enough for us to live well. We had other assets and investments, including properties that I hoped could appreciate in value and be converted to cash someday. I congratulated myself when I made periodic financial statements. I started to think of the possibility of being rich.

The real estate business has no institutional memory. Only the crudest statistics are kept regularly, so it is impossible to tell, except retrospectively, when a downturn, a sluggish period, or a crash, occurs. That knowledge is further deferred by the furious denial engaged in by the people in the business who want the good times to last forever. I knew the good times were over in about 1987, but I was dead wrong about how long it would take for even a weak recovery to begin. I earned no new income for about six years, living entirely from investments and dipping into savings. Toward the end of that time the leases on the income properties we had bought for investment ran out and we could not re-lease them for rents that would even pay the mortgage. We lost them. The only one left, and the most significant, was the Circle K. Now they were telling me in a letter that I could either accept half the rent or receive nothing.

Because the letter from Circle K had arrived while I was still in New Haven, I thought I had better visit the site before I responded: to have it fresh in mind to be better able to negotiate. I envisioned the brisk traffic I would see in the store and at the gas pumps. When I saw it I was horrified. Without giving me a chance to negotiate they had moved out of the building, stripped it clean, and even removed the gas pumps. Most of what they had taken did not even belong to them. The site looked desolate. The early signs of vandalism were in evidence.

I crept back to my office, feeling beaten, afraid and poor. I couldn't help wondering whether there would have been a different outcome had I been in town to receive their letter instead of being with Marty. The gods had been malevolent. They had drawn me out of town rendering me unable to defend my interests and then given no weight at all to my meritorious behavior. Not only would we have no income but it would cost plenty to recover the equipment Circle K had taken, and without it there was no hope of finding another tenant. I was sitting in my office, staring out the window aimlessly, plummeting into despondency. Soon we would consume our life savings and wouldn't be able to meet our expenses. We wouldn't be able to afford our house. Bill collectors would start to hound me, an experience I thought I had seen the last of twenty years before. We wouldn't have the funds to help our kids should they need it. I would be taken into the village square, stripped and beaten unmercifully in front of people I thought were friends, who would exult in my undoing.

A smile formed, not only on my face but somewhere inside, letting the wild exaggeration settle. Nothing of the sort was going to befall us. This was a setback, and coming at this time, a serious one. The real difficulty was that at that moment, not able to think of much else but Marty, I didn't feel the motivation to attack this business matter with the drive that I knew it would take to successfully rescue the situation. I would have to drum up the strength, the concentration.

I decided to try a technique to reduce stress that I had read about in a book, called, engagingly, "Full Catastrophe Living", by a friend of Marty's, Jon Kabott-Zinn. Marty had taken his course in stress reduction and found it helpful. I sat up straight-backed in my chair, fixed on a point across the room with half opened eyes and breathed deeply from the belly for five minutes or so. Somewhat calmed, feeling a respite from the panic overtaking me, I could begin to think through the gloom. I didn't realize it at the time but it was the beginning of my interest and practice of meditation. Resolving to use the breathing exercise regularly, I made a list of things that needed to be done immediately, complete with time schedules and phone numbers. And then I went to work. We would not be poor. We would be just fine. Marty will survive. We'll see to it. I'll see to it.

Marty struggled to regain his strength. Even after he returned from the hospital he was in distress for much of the time. Fatigued and still in considerable pain, he was in doubt as to which direction his health was heading. The medical indications showed that he was recovering well from the splenectomy, perhaps even recovered. His body told him otherwise. Stooped with pain, he dragged himself around his house, hoping to soon be ready to initiate the chemotherapy and on to the BMT. The winter was cold. Even inside his house, he found it hard to stay warm. He went back to the hospital a short time later with a stomach ailment the doctors could not identify.

When I spoke to Marty by telephone I could sense that he hoisted his spirits up higher than he felt so that I would not become discouraged. He knew how frustrating it would be for me to hear a bad report without being able to see him. Even so, I detected an increasingly flatter tone to his voice. It was a voice he could not have wanted anyone to hear but he was losing control over his ability to conceal it. I couldn't put a name to it at the time, but he was becoming depressed, a condition much more serious than I had ever understood. I feared for Vilunya. Marty could not hide his pain and the lowering of his spirits from her. The times I spoke to her, every third or fourth call to Marty, I could hear how frayed she was becoming. Once, in response to my question, really a pre-symbolic utterance, "How are you", she paused for a good while to let the catch in her throat relax somewhat and replied, "Lately, when I hear that question, I feel like crying."

At nineteen, when I was living in California in what would now be described as a commune, I returned to New York, to Brooklyn, in January, on a whim, for a visit. I traveled by Greyhound bus without telling anyone I was coming. Marty was living at home and going to City College, before his army service. I had no clear purpose in coming home, no fixed length of stay in mind. I hadn't seen my parents or Marty in over a year and I had seldom written. For the first couple of weeks the visit was pleasant; catching up on the time we hadn't seen each other. Marty and I slept in the same bedroom we shared as children, the same beds a couple of feet apart, surrounded by the same pieces of yellowish, curly maple furniture, bearing the scars of our childhood battles. Although neither one of us could articulate it, we both felt ourselves being sucked into the old, oppressive pattern. One morning, after I had been home a couple of weeks, we woke up and looked at each other sadly. Marty said to me, "I'll walk you to the subway." That was all. There was no further discussion. We both knew it had to be. As soon as I could say goodbye to our parents we left.

We set out on that cold Brooklyn winter morning, turning from Crown Street into the full winter wind along Troy Avenue, a route we had trod many, many times. Walking past all too familiar landmarks, hands deep in pockets, bodies tensed against the tearing wind and cold. With little conversation and hardly noticing the stores we walked past, the tiny stores, the puny enterprises, home and business to neighborhood families, we trudged on unwillingly, weighed down with inevitability. The stores, on street level, with apartment houses rising from them, looking like they were being crushed by the weight of the stone and brick on top of them, seemed insignificant yet necessary in the neighborhood. In every block or two they were duplicated; a fruit and vegetable and fish market, grocery store, candy store (luncheonette), drug store, tailor shop, shoemaker, butcher. Each household shopped at specific stores, usually the closest ones. We brushed along them, staring at the ground, dodging around occasional piles of gray snow lying in the shade of the buildings, not letting the wind find a vulnerable spot in our defenses, aware of the uniqueness of each store by smell or sound and peripheral vision. Our senses, conditioned from childhood, told us of the warm comfort of coffee from the candy store, sour pickle and cheese from the grocery, the gentle, rhythmic hammering wafting on the strong smell of leather and glue from the shoemaker's, the classical music that crept out of the underlit sanctum of the tailor's, the muscular smell of fish from the live fish tank in the vegetable store and fish market, especially when the stocky, powerful, old woman, dressed in many layers of clothing, wrestled a two foot long fish out of the tank, clubbed it to death on the weathered and scarred board, gutted, scaled and sliced or filleted it for customers, the drug store, whose window revealed little of the power of the potions contained in the floor to ceiling aged, dusty shelves or the butcher, who could be seen from between the hanging pieces of meat in his window, insouciantly sharpening his dangerous knife rapidly on a steel, looking ninety degrees away, to the street.

The proprietors were not simply merchants. They were experts: just enough chocolate syrup in the egg cream, not the hint of a rough edge along the new sole, careful, orderly, stitches on the altered garment, pickles that shriveled the inside of the mouth and at the same time refreshed it with garlic and spices, the surety of convincing a customer of the advisability of a patent medicine or of the necessity of consulting a doctor.

We broke our silence when we reached the vast boulevard, Eastern Parkway, on which the subway entrance coldly loomed.

"What time does your bus leave?"

"I don't know."

"You didn't call for a schedule?"

"No."

"How do you know you won't have to wait a long time?"

"I don't know. I probably won't. There probably are lots of buses going to California."

"You want me to come and wait with you, keep you company?"

We looked at each other furtively, but with eyes hungrily recording these last pained moments, the dark subway entrance gaping nearby.

"No, it's time to go."

"I know."

We waved goodbye, standing about ten feet apart. Handshaking or embracing each other was unknown to us in those days. A wave usually indicated that we would see each other shortly, although we had no idea when that would be. It turned out to be more than two years. Marty was standing at the top of the stairs, the bright, unforgiving, winter light silhouetting him, etching his forced, sad, smile in my memory, while I, unable to understand the turmoil I was feeling, was standing in the transitional light, the fading natural light blending with the decadently artificial yellow illumination underground. A dizzy hollowness surrounded us as we knew we had to part once again. We were certain of that without knowing precisely why. Caught in that feeling of sick emptiness, we lingered a moment, frozen, a hand in the air, eyes fastened on the other, before Marty turned to walk home and resume his life and I descended further underground to take the train to the bus terminal and return to California, each of us a little relieved that the parting was accomplished and we could be alone while the ache subsided.

Over the next few weeks Marty seemed to improve. His pain was diminishing and gradually he was getting stronger. More importantly, he was becoming convinced of his recovery from the splenectomy and interested in taking the next step, the chemotherapy, as soon as possible. His platelet count had moderated. He developed no new infections. He even put on a few pounds. Our communication, by telephone, had reached a calmer state. Our conversation almost invariably centered on his health, which he summarized briefly at the beginning of most calls. I liked it that way. The maintenance quality, the summing up of events transpired since our last talk, gave a feeling of normalcy to the situation, which in turn, quieted my guilt over not devoting more thought to Marty.

I was slowly working out my business problems. I was negotiating a lease with a new tenant. Even at a little more than half the rent of the old lease, I was grateful for the prospect of rescuing the property. What could have upset the entire plan was that it appeared that a gasoline tank might have sprung an undetected leak and contaminated the site. The court had permitted the bankrupt tenant to be absolved of any responsibility for environmental cleanup. It was therefore possible that I could have been forced to spend so much for the cleanup that I could have been drained of assets I had worked all my life to accumulate. Although I clung to an optimistic common sense belief that such an unfair outcome was improbable, if not impossible, the more I learned about this new subject the more I heard of examples of just such a result and the more frightened I became. I determined that this was a financial life threatening problem that had to be addressed carefully, methodically, step by painstaking step. The trouble was that every time I had to think through an aspect of the problem to arrive at a decision, my mind would begin to run amuck. I would conjure up the many pitfalls of making an incorrect move and would imagine the punishments that would be visited upon me for making such a mistake. There were no subtleties in those fantasies. Financial ruin was one of the swiftest consequences as well as my wife's loss of respect for me for having ruined our family. Although I believed I was slogging through my business problems somewhat satisfactorily, the process was draining me. I didn't have much energy left for Marty, or indeed, much of anything else. I decided to further explore meditation.

Marty first encountered meditation in the course on stress reduction he took with Jon Kabot-Zinn. A series of tapes came with the course. One part of the tapes was a series of guided yoga exercises. The other explored the rudiments of meditation. Primarily of interest to Marty was what was called a body scan. Concentration, through breathing, was brought to bear on various parts of the body. Marty benefited from this exercise whenever he did it. It was easy to do. One would lie down in a comfortable position with Jon Kabot-Zinn's soothing voice gently directing the thoughts and movements involved in the body scan. It was non-threatening, non-demanding and it left me with a calm, relaxed feeling. For Marty it helped control his physical pain.

I had by now started to read about what was beginning to be commonly referred to as the mind/body connection. While some of the claims seemed exaggerated to me, the essential aspects of it had the virtue of common sense. Evidence was mounting toward the conclusion that prolonged stress weakens the immune system, making one more susceptible to disease. While the evidence was largely anecdotal, and while many people in the field had questionable or no credentials, traditional scientists, some of great repute, were beginning to become interested. A field of study known as psychoneuroimmunology was developing. Jon Kabot-Zinn, for example, was a microbiologist before he began devoting all his time to instructing people in meditation for the purpose of reducing stress. Instinctively I believed that stress is destructive to the human organism. At least I felt it was having a bad effect on me and I did not doubt that I would be subject to more stress for a more extended period of time than ever before. I felt it was hurting me, was distorting and weakening me.

If that formulation was true, the reverse of it stood a good chance of being true, that is, reducing stress could strengthen the immune system. Numerous studies and experiments showed how altering the state of mind could affect physical response, such as respiration being affected by bio-feedback. I had always been curious about meditation and now seemed the perfect time to try it. Years before, when Transcendental Meditation swept the country I knew many people who tried it. I did not. At the time it seemed too voguish and I didn't have the $125 to lay out for a mantra. Everyone I spoke to who had tried it, without exception, said it made them feel calmer, less anxious. Everyone, also without exception, gave up the practice after a few months.

I knew that I had to be as healthy as possible to be of maximum use to Marty for the bone marrow transplant. After years of putting it off I scheduled an operation to have a bone spur removed from my big toe. Meditation, exercise, eating a healthy diet, were all part of my program to arrive at the transplant in the best shape I'd been in years. Marty would have the best marrow I was capable of giving him.

Alone, early in the morning, I would sit quietly, with earphones, listening to Jon Kabbat-Zinn's calm, measured voice, exhorting me to do something that had sounded difficult and somewhat foolish until I actually began doing it. After some weeks it felt less suspect and within a short time after that, I felt comfortable doing it and could experience its benefits. Kabot-Zinn talked of mindfulness. By that he meant being aware of what was occurring moment by moment and acting with that awareness. As I read more about meditation, I realized that his line of teaching came from a strain of Buddhism called Vipassana. I wasn't trying to become a Buddhist. I just wanted to learn how to meditate. At the moment I didn't aspire to more than taking myself in tow.

Early in my reading I was struck, almost physically, for the second time in my life, by the power of something I had read: the immediate, said by a Zen commentator was that the two principal bars to living in the present are regrets about the past and fear for the future. That could not have been truer of me. One or the other of those strong reactions would almost inevitably appear when I was in a stressful state and had to arrive at a decision, threatening to crowd out my ability to think clearly. If meditation, from whatever discipline it came, could help achieve the goal of living in the present without being assailed by specters of the past or future, I was all for it.

The first was when Jonathan was born. Two weeks after fleeing from the Malibu fire along with wild-eyed, sweat-glistening horses freed from burnt corrals, field rats as big as dogs driven from their wooded haunts by flames that licked the escaping car, Jonathan was born.

He came at one o'clock in the morning after a labor that lasted 12 or 13 hours. I saw him being born. I held him. The nurse took Jonathan away to allow Arline some sleep and I sat with her for a few minutes looking at her perspiration glowing face, more radiant and holy than any Renaissance depiction of a saint. We exchanged words of love and she bade me get some rest before she fell sweetly off to sleep, almost in the middle of a sentence. I left the hospital and began walking, surrounded by silence and the still, cool, night air.

I was a changed person, at twenty-two a boy no longer. The lights from the heavens affirmed it. The sound of my shoes striking the pavement affirmed it. I was strong and capable, loved by a beautiful woman, daddy to a new son. Whatever I had done before then, wherever I had been, what thoughts and plans and speculations about the future were now rendered provisional and non binding. The world's future, all history, would now begin. And then I remembered that Miguel de Unumuno had said in The Tragic Sense of Life that when your first child is born you get a glimpse of both your own immortality and of the grave.

Marty began chemotherapy March 25th. His new drug protocol was called DHAP, consisting of Dexamethasin, high dose Ara-C (Cytarabine Arabasine) and Cysplatin. Prior to beginning this first round Marty developed a sinus infection, something we thought he was through with as a result of the surgery he had had the year before. A new sinus expert was called in. More tests were administered. More tests were recommended. More surgery was discussed. The same caution from a year ago was repeated about the dangers that sinusitis would present to Marty after his immune system was further impaired by the chemotherapy. Finally, Dr. Rappeport said, in a statement worthy of a healer, "You are more than a sinus" and approved the beginning of chemotherapy. Salvage chemotherapy, the doctors called it.

The theory was that with the removal of his spleen, Marty would no longer be "refractory" to the chemotherapy, that is, the chemotherapy would now work to prepare him for the bone marrow transplant. Marty's white blood count was 200,000 and his platelet count was normal. Within two weeks his white count was less than 100,000 and he was sick with all the effects of the chemotherapy. It was good news, even for Marty, who knew he was going to get sicker and weaker. For the next four months, through three more rounds of chemotherapy, as the toxins accomplished their purpose, Marty sank lower and lower, at least twice having symptoms that could have killed him.

He was admitted to the hospital in mid-May with a high fever. I spoke to him a day or two before he was admitted. He was in bad shape. His back was aching and he couldn't move without extreme pain. He sounded very nasal, giving rise to the fear about the return of the sinus infection. He couldn't talk much. He gave the phone to Vilunya, who sounded on the verge of panic. She told me she "wasn't ready for this." When I called the next day Vilunya, sounding better than she had in days, told me that Marty was in the hospital, where a medical emergency could be attended to. They gave him the third round of chemotherapy days after his several days in the hospital.

Rappeport was pleased with the results. His white count was down below 50,000. A CAT scan showed that his lymph nodes were shrinking. He was going to think about whether to give Marty a fourth round. He said he "wanted Marty to be in the best condition for the transplant." I made plans to visit him in mid June.

Several days before I was to leave, during an examination with his doctor, Marty started trembling and grew too weak to support himself. His temperature was 103. The doctor admitted him to the hospital immediately with instructions for him not to be allowed even to go to the bathroom by himself. Marty's platelet count was 9,000, so low that the doctor feared that if Marty bumped against something hard or fell, he would start bleeding, possibly uncontrollably. I spoke to him the next day, a day before I was scheduled to leave to see him. We spoke for a minute or so. He said he wasn't doing too well, that he had a "little pneumonia." He was unable to talk more.

I went straight from the airport to Mount Auburn, a suburban hospital of perhaps two hundred beds. The contrast between it and the Yale Medical Center was startling. I walked through a clean, well-furnished lobby: carpets that showed no holes or stains, walls that were not scuffed or gouged. The few people sitting around were speaking quietly. The elevators, the halls, the waiting rooms and later, the patient's rooms, all seemed larger, calmer, neater, more respectful of illness.

Marty was sitting up in bed, looking expectant and brighter than I imagined he would be. Even allowing for some acting it was apparent he was feeling better than when I had spoken to him last. He had a large, private corner room overlooking the Charles River. His "little pneumonia" was yielding to antibiotics. He had received transfusions of both platelets and whole blood. The effect was dramatic. His platelet count rose immediately, but was still dangerously low at 28,000. The transfusions perked him up like a spring tonic. Even so, he was too weak to stroll the corridors and he was still throwing up regularly. It seemed clear he was going to make it through this latest episode but it was too early for him to go home. He remained in the hospital throughout my visit, comfortable and safe and glad to be that way for the first time in months. I stayed with him during the days, and late one evening to watch the basketball finals. During the days we talked, lightheartedly for the most part. I met friends of his who came by to visit. Nate, whom I hadn't seen since the previous fall, came every day.

It was pleasant sitting in his cheerful hospital room, visiting, chatting, exchanging small talk with his visitors, listening to the subjects of current interest to Marty's friends and colleagues. All the signs of normalcy were in evidence to the unknowing eye. Marty, looking artificially robust, displayed all the signs of a person recovering from a minor ailment, anticipating being discharged in a day or two to resume a completely normal life. His white blood count had come down from over 200,000 to about 10,000. Even with the platelet transfusions he had little clotting ability. All indications were that his immune system was shot, unable to defend his body from opportunistic infection. And they were planning to give him one more round of chemotherapy, on July 6th, a little more than two weeks from the time I saw him in the hospital. I returned home to try to resume a normal life for a while.

The date for the transplant was set. Marty would be admitted to the hospital August 5, 1993. I would travel from Phoenix and join him there later that same day and in the course of that month we would know if he would live or not. The month of July would be a hard one for everyone. Marty had to hang on, to fight the therapeutic poisoning he was undergoing, and to stay alive until the transplant. The rest of us had to remain steady. For me that meant not to let the morbid thoughts that seared my mind spill out in my conversations with Marty.

Some months before Marty had sent me a book about the Bone Marrow Transplant unit at the Yale Medical Center and Doctor Rappeport. What was supposed to tie the book together was a series of vignettes about various transplantees, written by a journalist whose sister had been a patient of Dr. Rappeport's. I thought it not a good book, because it reached for easy sympathies, more a series of magazine stories than a cohesive book. What struck me most was that, although her sister died, she never confronted it in her book. She dwelt on the process and on the outcomes of the other patients, but just mentioned, almost in passing, her sister's death. In a way I understood how that could happen. How can art be made of consuming personal tragedy? How hard it is to express the pain of losing a sibling, or in my case, my twin brother.

Another book I read about a bone marrow transplant involved a priest in Massachusetts, a man about our age. A frank, straightforward book, revealing the difficulty of facing what we were about to face, even though he was armed with belief in God. The priest let the writer into his life, discussed all manner of subjects with him, including sexual indiscretions that took place shortly after he was ordained and how that experience forced him to choose for life whether he took his calling seriously. The portrait that emerged was of a man who understood how difficult life was and who faced it without fear or unrealistic expectations. He ministered to his parishioners with blunt talk tempered with ready forgiveness for human faults. He wavered on matters of dogma but insisted on people conducting their lives with decency. He spoke of his leukemia the way one would expect of a priest. He would struggle against the disease but in the end his fate would be in higher hands and he would submit peacefully, graced by his belief.

He survived the transplant but was left with graft versus host disease. GVHD is caused by the match of the bone marrow not being quite close enough between the donor and the recipient. The recipient, the host, identifies the donated or grafted marrow as a foreign substance and tries to kill it. The symptoms that struggle produces can be horrible and the consequences fatal. He suffered so, he told his interviewer, that had he known how bad it was going to be he would not have had the transplant.

He would have chosen death. His suffering made him abdicate his faith, a denial of the meaning of his life.

It made me understand, in a way that none of the technical reading I had done for the past couple of years was able to do, what torments might lay ahead for Marty. I never told him of the book.

I plunged into my work, eager to be occupied with activities that could draw my thoughts away from Marty and the BMT, at least temporarily. With a little over a month to go life seemed unbearably complicated. How could I accomplish everything I had to in that time?

It was particularly hot in that Phoenix July, day after day 110 degrees and above. I was spending a lot of time outdoors testing the gasoline tank suspected of leaking at the convenience market. My toe, after the bone spur removal, felt worse than it did before. My son and his wife were expecting their first child in late July, and I knew I wouldn't be able to see them until after the transplant. The plan was that Arline would go to Cincinnati shortly after the baby came, spend some days there and join me in New Haven. She would return to Cincinnati after the transplant and I would meet her there, on the way home. I had to make the arrangements for a place to stay for the month in New Haven and conduct a rather bizarre negotiation with my health care insurer as well as with the hospital.

None of these problems individually would have daunted me, not even the potentially ruinous gas tank situation, but with the transplant looming I found it excruciatingly difficult to make even the simplest arrangements, or in the case of the gas tank, the complicated decisions. It was as if these acts, these simple arrangements became talismanic events. If, for instance, I never booked a hotel room in New Haven I wouldn't be able to go and, as a result, there couldn't be a transplant. If there couldn't be a transplant, Marty couldn't die. My rational, realistic thinking never got beyond that formulation. Marty would just exist in that condition, in that intermediate state, somewhere between health and the painful process he was facing. He wouldn't have to suffer and I would not be forced to think about it.

I did indeed make the necessary arrangements. Before I booked my flight however, I called the hospital to find out exactly what day they wanted me to be there. I was planning on being away about thirty days, more if needed. My inclination was to arrive as late in the process as I could so that I would be sure to be present when the success of the procedure would be apparent. My fantasy was of being there until he was fully recovered and able to go home. I pictured the drive back to Lexington, just like after the splenectomy some seven months earlier. I was told that the transplant was scheduled for August 12th. I was advised to arrive perhaps a day earlier, if that was convenient. I thought it over for a while and called back.

"You told me to be at the hospital the 12th or the 11th."

"Right."

"Martin will be admitted the 5th and begin the conditioning regimen which will involve intensive radiation and chemotherapy. Do I have that right?"

"That's correct."

"After the chemotherapy and radiation he'll have no ability to fight infection, he'll have no immune system. Is that right?"

"Yes."

"What happens if I get killed or for any other reason fail to show up at the hospital after you've given him those treatments? He'll surely die, won't he?"

"Very likely."

"Wouldn't it more advisable if I appeared at the hospital on the 5th?"

"Yes, that would be much better. Could you do that?"

I made the reservation for the 5th.

Our first grandchild was born on July 25th, 1993, in Cincinnati. Asa was the first born son of a first born son of a first born son. I hadn't thought about that until Arline pointed it out to me, but as I considered it, I was filled with wonder. And also a sad dread that I couldn't immediately discover the reason for. The awful comparison then came to me. As our father lay dying in a Los Angeles hospital, eleven years before, my nephew Ben, Phil and Joy's son, was being born in the same hospital. I couldn't help connect the two circumstances. Dad remained alive for about six weeks after Ben's birth. Although they never saw each other, and were separated by eighty-six years, the blood connection between the two of them weighed on us all with sadness, diluting what should have been the joy of welcoming a new child into our family.

The comparison was faulty, I told myself. Marty was not Asa's grandfather. They will not be in the same hospital, much less the same city. Marty was not eighty-six. But I could not help thinking of the terrible similarities. My thoughts, contorted by fear and stress, placed Marty and me and our whole family, in a mythic tide, moved by irresistible forces. The old must die so the young can live. Fair or not, that was the cosmic bargain. I started imagining the life leaking out of Marty as Asa grew stronger and gained a more secure purchase on life. When I would catch myself spinning these thoughts out with greater and greater detail I would angrily denounce myself for a fool and a coward for fleeing into fantasy to escape the necessary business of preparation for the transplant. Wherever I was I would try to rid myself of the debilitating mood with breathing exercises, a truncated meditation. Sometimes it worked.

I arranged my business matters, with the exception of the leaking gasoline tank, so that they could be taken care of by others in my absence, with an occasional phone call from me from New Haven. I temporarily resolved the gasoline tank matter by signing a contract to have it removed from the ground. That would insure that nothing needed to be done till I returned and at least I could try not to worry about it while I was gone. When I returned to Phoenix I would know the extent of the contamination and how long and how much it would take to remediate. It worried me more than I would admit.

Until my departure from Phoenix I saw my task as staying calm and remaining healthy. I tried to do everything possible to allay fear and panic. Daily meditation became an increasingly comfortable practice. I visited a dermatologist to have him look at a minor skin break that I thought was not healing, thinking of the remote possibility of it being a fungal infection, something I thought to be dangerous if transmitted to Marty. The doctor looked at me as if I were crazy and gave me a topical salve to apply to it. It vanished in a day or so.

Arline left for Cincinnati a few days before I left for New Haven. We spoke on the phone daily. She was purring with happiness at seeing and holding her first grandchild. She told me in detail how beautiful he was, how outstanding his every physical characteristic. I heard his infant squeal. I carried his picture around with me, stealing glances at it, feeling strengthened by the sight of the little fellow.

Now that I could see him, my tiny grandson, and hear him described by Arline and hear the fatigued wonder and exhilaration in the voices of Diane, his mother, and Jonathan, my earlier fearful formulation changed completely. Rather than Asa's arrival being the trade for Marty's demise, the bawling battle to survive and to grow that Asa was beginning would somehow nourish Marty, would help him in his struggle to survive. Asa was one more soldier in Marty's army. I felt stronger and more clear-headed than I had in some time. I would arrive in New Haven ready to help in the battle.

A couple of days before my departure I was called by a woman with an Italian surname who worked in the business office of the Yale-New Haven Medical Center. After she verified who I was and that I was to be the donor in Marty's bone marrow transplant, she asked me for my health insurance information. I was somewhat puzzled and asked her why my health insurance was involved. She told me that Marty's health insurance might not cover the cost of the donor. I was dumbfounded. I asked her to please explain to me how a bone marrow transplant was able to be achieved without the donation of the bone marrow, and hence, without the donor. And, wasn't it a little late in the day to be finding out about this important detail? Slowly, and with kindness, she explained to me that the procedure that had to be followed was to ask my insurance carrier to pay for my participation in the BMT and, when, predictably, they refuse, Marty's carrier would pay for it. Her voice indicated that she thought it was as crazy as I did. I imagined her as a plump, middle-aged, olive-skinned dumpling, with gray glistening through her black hair, her quick, chocolate brown eyes sighting her interviewee down her long nose. I met her several days later at the hospital. Although it was obvious she didn't remember me, she did indeed look as I had pictured her. At that time I found out that my insurance company had refused to pay and Marty's had agreed to, exactly as she had predicted.

Marty had been lying low the last few weeks, preparing himself for the BMT. He sent the following letter to some 120 friends and colleagues;

July 28, 1993
Dear ,

On August 5th I am scheduled to enter Yale-New Haven Hospital to undergo a bone marrow transplant (BMT) to hopefully cure the chronic lymphocytic leukemia (CLL) I have had for almost 22 years. Although we had made the decision to have the BMT in February 1992, the road to August 5th 1993 has been torturous, difficult and enlightening.

I completed the spring semester '92 with some difficulty, that included a sinus operation, and immediately started a program of chemotherapy to reduce the burden of my CLL and improve my chances of success in the BMT. I underwent two different chemo regimens (CHOP, Fludarabine) neither of which seemed to work, i.e. my spleen and lymph nodes continued to enlarge. My doctor at that time thought that a splenectomy might help (although he wasn't sure). That was October '92 and I spent the rest of that month studying my situation and arranging to have the splenectomy done in Yale-New Haven Hospital. That meant getting my health plan to agree to do this out of state (no small job).

I entered the hospital on November 30th for the surgery that was supposed to take about a week. Possibly because of the size of my spleen, (larger than most babies), I had to be reoperated to stop massive bleeding, and spent time in intensive care. I got out about 17th and four days later had to be shipped back there for a thrombosis of a large vein in my abdomen. That stay lasted another two weeks.

After a three months recovery from that, involving a hospitalization for a mysterious stomach ailment, I began a round of "salvage" chemotherapy. Medical poetics (the language doctors use with each other) are crystal clear as opposed to medical euphemisms (the sweet talk doctors use with patients to avoid unpleasantries like pain and suffering). This chemo worked well. Each of the four monthly rounds brought my blood counts down and reduced the portion of my blood taken up by leukemic cells. Working well also came to mean that I got sicker and sicker, requiring two hospitalizations for the complications they produced.

So I am now as "tumor free" as can be hoped for and ready for the transplant. The transplant process involves first destroying my marrow, and therefore my immune system, with radiation and chemotherapy. That takes about a week and when it is done, I'll receive the marrow given by my identical twin brother Saul. The weeks without an immune system are the most dangerous part with the greatest risk of dying from uncontrollable infection. An identical twin donor eliminates the other risk, chronic graft-versus-host disease, a sequel to transplant that can itself involve a life-long illness.

Saul will come to New Haven from Phoenix and stay there until I am out of the woods. Vilunya, Leah and Aaron, having lived through this with me, are ready. Leah has been living with us since last fall, experiencing the rough spots and helping us through them. Aaron has been away at school, but home for the Summer, and grappling with these difficulties. The past fourteen months have transformed us as a family. We've been compelled to face the possibility of my death and its meaning for each of us. Vilunya has responded so fully and lovingly that it seems inconceivable for me to be at my present point without her good cheer and companionship. Leah and Aaron have each evolved in this situation in a way that has accelerated their development. My disease has been an intrusive companion for years but, being incurable (except for a transplant), it now forces us all to think about mortality and its meaning for us as a family.

For me, the disease has permitted me to live fairly normally for twenty of the past twenty-two years. During that time I have moved from feelings of fragility and terror to a state of awareness of the tenuousness and transience of life in general. My first hematologist, a man of few words, counseled me to "make plans" and that is what I have tried to do.

Since my disease became intractable, about two years ago, most of my planning has been about the different therapies and medical responses suggested by the doctors. This has taught me several things. First, that I can be active in deciding on medical options that affect me. That active state of mind has given me strength and I feel has a healing impact. Second, I rebound quickly from the many medical insults (no euphemism) I've received. I don't require perfect health to feel alive, even optimistic. Third, if fighting against illness means anything, for me it means the clear sense that I still have much to do after my transplant. This presumption of survival leaves little room for dwelling on disaster and keeps me in touch with the larger issues that have always engaged me. These larger issues (social justice) reduce the impulse to feel that my problems are unique in the world.

When I recover from this ordeal, over the next year, it will be with a heightened sense of appreciation for all the small, quotidian events that make up the bulk of our lives. It will also help me place myself in context, to more fully use whatever capabilities I have acquired as academic, teacher, husband, parent and friend to the struggles that will outlive us all.

Your affection and support through these tough times have helped me maintain focus on the enduring qualities of one's life, a focus that will come in handy for my entire future.

Love,

Marty

That letter was not sent to me or even shown to me when it was mailed to Marty and Vilunya's friends. I found out about it later by happenstance, a remark made in my hearing referring to it. When I asked about it a copy was produced with the salutation, Dear Saul and Arline, written by hand on the Xeroxed copy of the typewritten letter. I didn't need the letter to know what had led to the transplant. I had experienced much of those events. It was a letter written to people who didn't know about either the transplant or the long illness that made it necessary, and who would certainly not play any part in it, a letter for colleagues, professional friends, acquaintances, not family or close friends, especially not for me. It enlisted the support and encouragement of those who received the letter, whose response would give Marty a therapeutic boost when he most needed it. It was clear, then, that it was not a letter for me.

And yet, it irritated me. Overall, it sounded to me like a sociology tract, full of academic descriptions of an intensely personal and frighteningly real situation. While I admired his bland understatement of his own suffering, I was annoyed at the description of his family's response to their crisis, especially at equating the response between Aaron and Leah. Aaron was being extremely difficult, giving both Marty, in his weakened state, and Vilunya, gut-grinding problems while Leah had sacrificed much to be of help.

I considered my irritation, embarrassedly. As I reviewed my list of complaints about style, purpose and content, I confessed that I was most put out over Marty's description of my participation. After hearing effusive expressions of praise and gratitude from doctors associated with Marty and words of admiration from friends of mine for what I had done and was about to do, I read his account of my participation merely as a description of one of a number of mechanical steps in the transplant instead of featuring me as the author of his salvation. I wanted a starring role. I wanted to hear paeans lavished upon me by Marty. I felt infantile as I spun out this line of thought, a boy back in the Brooklyn of the late 1940's. I was doing all this for him, without which he could not survive, and he was ranking me. What an affront. What a joke.

At six years old, Marty and I are thrilled to be in the midst of a battle involving the big boys. The battleground is a small milk delivery truck parked in the front of the six story walkup apartment house we live in. Several of the boys, twelve to fourteen years old, are installed defensively in the bed of the truck and a like number on the sidewalk try to storm the fortress. Marty and I excitedly enjoy the duel, happily jostled by both sides. Suddenly, I am seized by the truck defenders and turned into a battering ram. Two or three of them are swinging me by the legs into the besiegers. It is fun no longer. The concrete sidewalk is a few feet below my head and shoulders and all that prevents my collision with it is my utility as a weapon. The boys on the sidewalk, including Marty, are as terrified as I am, pushing me up, back toward the bed of the truck. All resistance to my fall stops and I am propelled toward the bare sidewalk, bulletlike, my hands at my sides. All goes blank. Nothing remains. Not even the sensation of pain.

I wake as I am borne by the boys up the stairs to our apartment. All have grave expressions at the sight of my bloody face. No serious damage results from the episode but for weeks after I am aware of the horror on the other mother's faces when they see the little boy whose face is covered in cuts and bruises.

Decades later, Marty told me he felt our mother blamed him for not preventing my injury. It surprised me. I thought it odd that he would harbor a thought like that for so long. Not that particular thought, but because I have my own inventory of such painful memories it made me understand that Marty and I will always feel the scars of ancient wounds, inflicted, according to the distortion of memory, either with the compliance of, or at the hands of, the other twin. Not the physical ones, whose presence can be proved by the finger brushing the depression of the long healed tear in the skin or the crooked broken finger or the slight asymmetry of the face never fully restored after a bad beating. In our own way those evidences of injury are pleasurable recollections, moments of action, of risk, of youth.

What we will always bear uneasily is the slight, the humiliation of the judgment that one of us was better than the other; smarter, stronger, more adept, destined to be more accomplished. Usually it was suffered at the hand of our father, sometimes unintentionally inflicted, sometimes deliberate. We always felt the bitter resentment toward the other, not against the parent who may have acted unfairly. We were always convinced that the other conspired in what we thought at the time was an injustice. As with all children, we wanted all our parent's love for ourself, even if it meant none for the other. At the same time each of us wanted his twin brother to defend him from defeat and humiliation at any cost, at any sacrifice, even the loss of parental love. To this day, even as men approaching old age, we can surprise the other with thoughts and memories of events that caused pain that the other had long forgotten or buried too deep to be conveniently retrieved. Perhaps it will always be so.

I was heavy and anxious as I left Phoenix. Leadenly dragging myself around the house, I tried to immerse myself in the myriad details involved in leaving for a month. I plodded through the paces of closing the house, trying to be deliberate about turning off those lights that should have been off, adjusting the thermostat correctly and carefully turning off the hoses watering the parched plantings. Those that I watered by hand would have to fend for themselves. If they were lucky there would be sufficient mid-summer rain to keep them alive. I obsessively inspected the door locks and the stove several times. At last the taxi arrived.

I thought of Marty on the plane. I tried to picture his precise circumstances. He had been admitted to the hospital the day before and by now was surely entombed in the sealed room he was to occupy until the transplant was over. My mind fled from a definition of "over". All I would allow was the happy thought of Marty leaving the hospital, cured.

Fortunately, no one sat next to me. My attempts at reading were a pretense. I was traveling with Marty, on the same journey. Every step each of us was taking was irrevocable. Marty was in his cabin, me in mine. He probably was gauging his progress by the various small, preparatory medical procedures he was undergoing. I was watching the fleece mountains of clouds drifting rapidly past the airplane, ticking off the distance between Marty and me. All the diagnosing had better be accurate, I thought, all the therapeutic strategy had better work out, or it will be the end of Marty, the end of the twins.

TRANSPLANT

To be in a reflective or self-pitying mood is not allowed in public in New York. The city wrenches you from that weakened condition and forces you to earn your living, your space on the sidewalk, your place on line, your right to demand that promises made be fulfilled. While I was waiting just outside of the terminal for the rental car agency van to pick me up a man sidled up to me and asked, in Spanish, if I wanted a ride into the city. I asked him if he was a taxi driver. Ignoring the question, he repeated his offer. Oddly warming to the exchange, I asked him how much it would be. He quoted me a price at least 25 percent higher than a metered cab. What an entrepreneurial city, I thought. This scam artist's niche was ferreting out Spanish speaking strangers to New York and fleecing them in their first economic encounter. I declined his offer as I climbed onto the van.

The neighborhood in which the car rental agency was located, near the airport, seemed a pleasant place as we drove through it. The large sycamores and elms, planted in orderly file at the edge of the street were in full leaf, permitting only scattered fingers of sunlight to prick the sidewalks underneath them. People were enjoying the warm, not overly humid weather. Life had spilled out of the single and two family houses, most of them attached to its identical neighbor. Children were playing everywhere. Women were sitting on chairs under the shade trees animatedly conversing, ostensibly watching their children. Men were gathered on the street corners lubricating their conversation with occasional sips from containers in paper bags. The neighborhood appeared to be inhabited by working people at their ease on a summer day, comfortable, safe and relaxed.

The van drove through a steel gate that opened in anticipation of its arrival and clanged shut as soon as it had entered. My driver vanished, leaving me to drag my luggage to the door of the office to discover that it was locked from the inside. A woman languorously made her way to the door, avoiding eye contact with me, undid the lock from the inside and without holding the door open for me, repaired to the bowels of the small, dirty office. I horsed the door open and deposited my bags on the floor. Although I was the only customer I was inexplicably made to wait until I asked that someone attend to me. The exchange was tedious. My ears still ringing from the airplane noise, I had to ask the young woman to repeat every *sotto voce*, heavily Caribbean accented question she asked me, then wait while her bored eyes tried to complete the typing on the form without breaking her garishly colored, inch long fingernails.

When the transaction was completed and the form signed, I asked her to direct me to the road that would take me ultimately to New Haven. She threw a map on the counter, and over her shoulder, told me to exit the yard, make a right, a left, get on a certain boulevard street and drive till I saw a sign to the something something parkway. If I had been there to transact business in New York, something I had done many times, and wanted to hone my actions and prepare my state of mind for the contentious days to follow, I would have made my stand there and then and demanded an explanation that satisfied me, no matter how long it would have taken. I didn't that day. I left the office defeated. I would stumble and bumble my way to the Hutchinson River Parkway and to the Merritt Parkway beyond. It was easier than beginning a fight I was in doubt about winning. Besides, I rationalized, I would need all my strength over the next month for more important battles.

It was dark when I arrived in New Haven. I checked into my extended stay hotel and immediately drove to the hospital, barely two miles away. Along the way, and as the streets began to look more familiar, recollected from my stay the previous December, I began to palpitate with anxious fear. At every step of the way over the past two years the thought existed that the great mistake would be discovered, that the awful dream would end, that Marty really did not have leukemia and would not need the transplant. But I would see him in a few minutes in his sealed enclosure and know beyond all controvertability that it was indeed so that his life was at stake. Parking in the lighted garage and retracing the steps I had taken last year nauseated me. I was sweating.

The unmarked Bone Marrow Transplant Unit was entered only from an unmarked door inside of a surgical ward, tucked away to discourage accidental traffic. I swung the large, portentous door open slowly, obeying the "open door carefully" sign. Another, larger, sign demanded that all entrants don paper booties over their shoes. I sat near the entrance, slipped on the booties and prepared myself to approach Marty's room.

We persuade Mommy and Daddy to let us stay alone one Sunday afternoon in mid winter. We are in first grade. They are going to visit friends, a childless couple they have known since before they were married. Marty and I dread having to sit around and be well behaved while our only recreation is listening to the adults drone on about things we can not understand and do not interest us.

Our real motive is not to miss listening to the radio program that both attracts and frightens us, The Shadow. The radio is still a great novelty for us. We aren't always permitted to listen to programs that entertain us and we know with certainty that there will be no chance if we go with our parents.

When we say our good-byes we promise not to let anyone in the apartment. We throw the deadbolt behind them as they bade us. The living room lights are not yet on. For economy, lights are never left burning needlessly nor turned on prematurely. If you can read with natural light, sitting near a window, so goes the unspoken rule, the electric lights are not needed.

Some dirty outside light still shines through the window near the upright radio set. As soon as we hear our parent's footfalls die away Marty and I bound about the living room trampolining on the overstuffed couch and chair, exulting in our freedom. We chase each other around the apartment, catching each other and roughhousing playfully. Our spirits are too high and our expectations too delicious to permit our horseplay to turn into a serious fight. Calming down, we decide to pass the time, almost an hour until the broadcast begins by playing Chinese checkers. One or the other of us looks at the clock in the kitchen every few minutes. Finally, unable to bear it any longer, about fifteen minutes before the broadcast we fly to the radio. One turns the ON dial while the other grasps the tuning dial awaiting the heating up of the tubes. Each gives commands to the other about how to operate his post. At last the station is found, broadcasting the silly serial immediately before The Shadow.

The radio stands at least as tall as we, a handsome, dark, wooded countenance, its important looking dials flanking the laminated wood filigree over the cloth that shields the speaker. It is a foot or two from the one window in the small living room which looks out on the brick and windows of the three other sides of the apartment building and the courtyard below. From where

Marty and I squat in front of the radio we see the frame through which the light appears to enter the room. From our angle the square window casement of our 5th floor apartment is slashed into a triangle by the roof parapet across the courtyard. Further encroaching on that space is the rounded top of the radio, so that the impression it gives is of a carefully marked path that the outside rays of moribund light follow, threading their way through a precise file of suspended dust motes.

At last the program begins. Almost as soon as we hear the dry, adult, unaccented, voice of the narrator describing how Lamont Cranston learned, in the Orient, the power to cloud men's minds so they could not see him, followed by the sinister, crackling laugh of the Shadow, Marty and I know we are trapped in the fear that quickly envelops us. For all we know the Shadow could be in the by-now darkened room with us. Not the justice-dispensing, kindly Shadow, but an evil one who would take pleasure in inflicting sadistic punishment on children without parents to defend them. We shrivel in fear, lying close to each other on the floor, at the foot of the imposing radio, the author of our torment. We do not cling to each other, both afraid to admit, even to himself, the degree of terror he is experiencing.

We can not move. We do not have a telephone to call for help, nor do we know how to use one. We have to endure our torture quietly. If we move too much the unseen forces surrounding us will surely assault us. Hunger does not budge us, or the urge to go to the bathroom. We can not walk across the small room to turn on a light. We lay in place until The Shadow ends. The news goes on, then a home improvement program, followed by a selection of dance music. And still we lay in place, only occasionally making small, grunting comments just to prove to ourselves that we are still alive and praying that the time will pass quickly till Mommy and Daddy return.

At last the key drills into the lock, turns the tumblers with the sound of an ax coming down a block of hard wood and the door, slightly stuck, yields and flies open with a bump of our father's shoulder. We jump to our feet, startled and relieved, snap the radio off and run to the door as our parents enter the pitch dark house.

"What's going on here? Why is it so dark?" says Dad as he turns the hall light on, smarting our eyes. We nestle into the embrace of their cold outer garments, pressing into them to savor the comforting smell of tobacco and our parents' bodies. Their faces are glowing with the outside cold.

As I stood up, both Marty and Vilunya saw me. Vilunya stood and blew me a kiss. His room was the second from the entry door. Vilunya was inside his room, fully swathed in surgical garb, including rubber gloves and face mask. I walked carefully, slowly, through the adjacent service room and stood not two feet from Marty separated by the plastic curtain wall. Marty smiled a relieved, sweet smile that masked the fear that could still be read in his face. We mumbled words of greeting. I felt the urge to say something clever, something funny. Nothing came except a stutter I could feel rising from my throat. Marty beckoned me to put my hand through the gauntlet that reached into his room through the plastic wall. I put both hands through and Marty grasped them. We stood, without speaking, looking at each other and holding hands. Vilunya looked on with gleaming eyes and cheeks bursting out of her surgical mask. I could not feel Marty, flesh to flesh. The touch of the plastic gauntlet felt repellent, now too cold, now slimily warm. It would have to do. No one would be able to touch him with an ungloved hand until he left his laminar flow room.

I felt the awful separation immediately. The real Marty was gone for the interim. He was traveling in the other country of his dual citizenship. Because he held valid passports in both lands he could stay in either one for as long as he wished, as long as was necessary. I understood that the person behind the plastic was corporeally Marty, but lacking the essence of Marty. He was a symbol of Marty, an echo, an approximation. Marty would be real again when he left the hospital. Leaving the hospital meant to me that he would be cured, the transplant a success. Until then I would have to settle for touching him through the plastic. I would have to accept hearing his muffled voice and seeing him somewhat distorted by the waves in the plastic. They would be indications of who he was; reminders of the real Marty. But for the moment the three of us were content, acknowledging that the process was finally begun, that Marty's walking store of marrow had arrived, that the last of his allies had arrived.

Vilunya left the room and embraced me through the scrub garments. While she changed I pulled a stool close to the plastic wall and Marty and I chatted somewhat nervously about my flight and hotel accommodations and about my first grandson, his grandnephew. A picture of newborn Asa, his face wrinkled in protest against some disturbance to his tranquillity, was pinned to the wall just outside the opening to the room, visible to Marty from his bed. Vilunya joined us minutes later and she and I repeated the conversation I had just had with Marty while he and I stole sly glances at each other.

Marty reclined in his bed at about forty five degrees while we talked. Penetrating the plastic wall were tubes that led from the I.V. stand, a device that looked like a hat rack, containing bottles of liquids to be given to Marty intravenously. The tubes led into one of the two Hickman catheters, surgically implanted in Marty's chest. Should it be needed, large quantities of medications could be given to him quickly. At the moment nothing was dripping through. By putting their arms through the plastic gauntlets the nurses could change the lines or clean the catheter or perform other tasks related to the I.V. system without having to enter the room.

Things were quiet in the Unit, as everyone called it. The other three patients had no visitors. Dinner had long since been over. The nurses were in their administrative core quietly doing paper work. The daylight had long since faded and the unsparing fluorescent light cast shadows over our faces. We talked softly, gradually introducing the subject of the days that would follow; the various procedures Marty would undergo leading to the transplant in seven days.

I left briefly to find a bathroom, passing two of the other three rooms. One of them was dark and the other dimly illuminated a young woman, sitting up in bed, watching television. She turned as she heard me pass and smiled at me, longingly, I thought. I returned the smile thinking that she mistook me for Marty, a familiar experience, until I realized that she probably had not met Marty, a prisoner for the time being like her. Carol was a twenty-eight-year-old woman from a nearby town, married, with two small children. One of her children, fifteen months old, was her donor. He was so small they had to harvest his marrow twice, about a month apart. I winced hearing that. The other two rooms were occupied by a Cambodian man in his forties, whom everyone called Pon, and Ray, a young, athletically built man of about thirty.

Over the next month I would have brief visits with Carol and Ray (Pon spoke no English) and daily exchanges with family members that came to visit them. These contacts were always shy and tentative on both sides, neither wanting to intrude upon the other, engaging only when it was clear beyond doubt that such attentions were welcome. Although at times, jokes and laughter were exchanged between the nurses and doctors and visiting family members and even patients, there was no levity between different patients' visitors. The brief conversations were always kind and respectful. The unit was a place of suffering and the closer you got to the plastic wall the more apparent it became. At times all visitors would look upon the misery of a beloved person, unable to help, the patient unable to conceal his pain. There would be many times when I wanted to bolt from the plastic wall and find a lighter environment, a meaningless conversation with a friendly stranger, a silly movie, a meal with shared gaiety. Several times I did leave, on some pretext, and usually walked outside the hospital till I regained my equanimity. Most of the time I waited until Marty fell asleep or had to have some procedure performed that required drawing his curtain. I was always aware, with an afflicted feeling, that I could leave but Marty could not.

I went to see Dr. Smith, a younger colleague of Dr. Rappeport. A large, fleshy, fair complected man in his middle forties, he conducted his business with me in an earnest manner. In this intake interview he gave me a brief physical exam and questioned me about my health. He paused, and looking directly at me, thanked me for being Marty's donor. I was nonplused. Didn't he know about twins? I was slightly embarrassed at the obvious sincerity of his statement. Just as it formed, a startled question came out of my mouth. "Do people who are well matched or identical to people with leukemia ever refuse to be their donors?" His eyes averted as he tried to disguise the weariness in his answer. "You'd be surprised."

In order not to forget them, and also to let him know the seriousness of my purpose, I opened the stenographers' pad I had written questions in, placed it on the edge of his desk and took the top off my ball point pen. He settled his bulky frame, letting me know that he was in no hurry. He tugged at his unruly hair as if trying to lift a patch of wild hair from one place on his scalp and place it on another, more appropriate, location. It was the gesture of a man who has much more important thoughts than of his hair, who defers forever finding the solution to eccentric, ill behaved hair. I liked the gesture. I liked the man. Leukemia was more important than hair.

"I'd like to know all about the transplant. The actual procedure, how long would it take for Marty to engraft. What would be the most dangerous time for him?" I paused, consulted my notes, giving him the option of answering questions piecemeal. I was determined that I wouldn't find myself out the door without having my questions answered.

"Any other questions? Perhaps the best way is to ask them all and talk about them. If any others occur to you I'll see if I can answer them."

"Good. What are the chances of affecting a cure? When can Marty go home? How long will it take for him to recover? How, physically, would the marrow get from me to Marty? How hard will the marrow harvest be on me?"

Dr. Smith made some sketchy notes as I asked my list of questions.

"Marty will, between now and the twelfth, six days from now, first be given aggressive chemotherapy and then full body radiation to completely destroy his sick marrow. The recent success of the 'conditioning' chemotherapy has increased the chances of killing all the leukemic cells. You will be admitted to the hospital the morning of the 12th and be prepared for the harvest. The marrow will be withdrawn from the large bones in your pelvic girdle, both front and back. A large needle will puncture the bone and marrow will be sucked out through the needle into the syringe. It is physically demanding on the doctors. Three of them will participate, myself, Dr. Rappeport and Dr. Ahmad, spelling each other as their hands and arms tire. We'll puncture the skin perhaps ten times and the bones perhaps one hundred and fifty to two hundred times. We'll withdraw about eight hundred CC's, approximately half the size of a large manila envelop bulging at the sides. Then, centrifuge out the bone chips and take the rest right to Martin. The marrow will be transfused, hung up on the I.V. stand and dripped through the Hickman. It will be in his body probably within two hours of the time it is withdrawn from you." He waited a moment while I made some notes. "It will probably take about three weeks for him to engraft."

Smith said that it would be hard to judge the chances for a cure. A very small population existed world wide of one of identical twins with chronic lymphacytic leukemia. The only one I had read the results of was a study done in France with some forty subjects. Smith's gross estimate was fifty-fifty for a cure. Even absent a cure, he was encouraging about the prospects of a major improvement, years and years - maybe ten years - of improved health.

Marty could be released from the hospital to begin his convalescence at home when his white count grew to an acceptable level and when his weight and appetite improved sufficiently. The most dangerous time for Marty, aside from the weeks without an immune system, would be the first hundred days or so after the transplant. His diet would have to be carefully controlled, and with the immune system of an infant, Pneumonia, and cytomegalovirus, would be two of the most extreme dangers. Others included a variety that ranged from liver damage to depression. Smith thought there was a 20% mortality danger in the transplant with a non perfect match. In Marty's case, with an identical march, he calculated the danger as less. Full recovery could take a year to eighteen months.

Brian Smith teaches, practices medicine and does research in immunology. He told me of his fascination with the similarities he has observed between the immune system and the neurological system. He guessed it will take forty years to uncover the relationship between the two. Realizing that any question I would ask about that subject would require a long answer, I did not pursue it.

Instead, I spoke of meditation and other techniques for relieving stress. Smith would not go further than volunteering his belief that relieving stress is a good thing. He did not disagree when I told him that I had formed the opinion from my reading that stress harms the immune system. Although I was left with the impression that he thought that the relationship between stress and the functioning of the immune system was a fruitful area of study, he was not going to show enthusiasm for such an unproved theory. I was pleased, though, that he did not give me the standard doctor's negative argument; that there was no certain relationship between stress and the immune system because there were no scientific studies that proved it. I would continue meditating no matter what he said.

We discussed the health care system. He, teacher, doctor and researcher and I, patient, consumer of medical services, agreed that reform was needed but would be tough to achieve. Smith suggested that while perhaps a 15 percent savings was possible through efficiency in administration the rest will take a change in the culture. By that I was sure he meant better preventative care, patients and doctors relying less on expensive diagnostic procedures and, in old age, not prolonging life as much as we presently do. While I agreed with it all, the last part of the formulation hit too close to home. Both my thoughts and speech were muted thinking of Marty who was, by the book, too old for the transplant he was about to have. Before it was finished the costs would probably reach $200,000, and would be "socialized" by increasing the insurance premiums on the rest of us. To hell with health care reform. Let it start right after Marty is cured.

After lunch I asked Marty if he felt like a visit in his room, on his side of the plastic. He welcomed it. Under the serious tutelage of Angela, one of the senior nurses, I scrubbed after changing into surgical garb. She stood at my side instructing me every step of the way. Several times she insisted that I repeat a certain operation. Considerably overweight, laboring in her movement about the unit, Angela was perhaps in her late fifties judging from the bulbousness in her face and the gray in her usually disheveled hair. Her luminescent bluish eyes invited a joke, a familiarity, while the steel in them indicated clearly that she was confident enough to set the limit. She made sure that I took the scrubup ritual seriously and admonished me to ask for help in scrubbing until I was expert at the task. Fully scrubbed, gowned, masked and gloved, I turned to enter Marty's room, excited at the prospect of seeing him without the distorting plastic for the first time. As I crossed the windy threshold of his room, still somewhat apprehensive that I might be transporting unseen contaminants, I discovered that he was fast asleep. I entered his room and sat down in a hospital version of an armchair to await his awakening and almost immediately fell into a deep sleep.

Over the next hour and a half Marty and I dozed and chatted intermittently. It was difficult for him to speak. Weak and nauseated, he was feeling the effects of the chemotherapy which had started that day with Cytosine Arabinoside (Ara-C). For the next few days Cyclophosphamide (Cytoxan) would be added. Early the following week and overlapping the end of the chemotherapy he would be given total body radiation twice a day. After that, purged of his own marrow, he would receive mine. At last, communicating with his deep brown eyes, moist with pain and fatigue, Marty let me know he could visit no longer today. I left to change clothes. When I returned three or four minutes later, Marty was asleep, his head sunken heavily in his pillows, his mouth slightly open.

Dr. Rappeport was standing behind me, quietly reviewing Marty's records. Not having seen him since the previous December I reintroduced myself. We left the immediate area so as not to disturb Marty with our conversation. Joel, as he asked to be called, ate a number of salt crackers and drank a cup of oily, burnt, coffee while we talked. Sprawled in a chair, he unselfconsciously rained crumbs on himself. I was spare with my comments and especially my questions, not wanting to drain the reservoir of answers too early in my stay.

Joel Rappeport never seemed to be moving toward a destination. He just filled a space the eye had observed as empty a moment earlier or glided around a corner and out of sight during a pause in conversation. Always leaning, drooping, hanging, he never moved quickly. His Levantine features and deliberate speech conveyed a languor that masked his essential restlessness. His eyes seldom fixed on the person he was speaking to, but neither did they dart around. Rather, he seemed to strain to capture yet one more degree of the periphery of vision so that he would not be denied all the information possible at the moment. During the month I spent in the hospital, having almost daily contact with him, I formed the opinion that he did not see his patient's illnesses as something static, but as a dynamic process, changing without warning or notice. In order to take care of them properly he had to review their progress day by day, sometimes hour by hour, especially the transplantees, to be able to respond to changes that, unchecked, could kill them.

To break the silence that was settling in, I told Joel of the phone call I had had from the business office asking if I had insurance. He livened up immediately.

"Yes, I heard about that too."

"I thought it kind of odd coming so close to the time of the transplant."

"I still have to write letters about it. That's what I have to do when I leave here tonight."

"But I received a notice, just like the woman in the business office said I would, that my insurance company refused to cover it and Marty's health plan has approved it."

"You got a written notice that it's been done?"

"Yes."

"Am I glad I ran into you," said Rappeport, brightening considerably. "That saves me about an hour of work tonight."

Although I had planned to buy some food that I could keep in the small kitchen of the hotel room, all I had succeeded in acquiring so far was a quart of gin. For those first nights, I returned to the hotel exhausted, poured a generous drink and plopped down in front of the television set to catch the news and remain glassyeyed, sometimes for an hour, before I'd stir to refill my glass. Usually I had phone calls to answer: Arline from Cincinnati, friends from Phoenix offering support and calls from Mom and Phil from Los Angeles.

I began to understand the obligation of the afflicted toward the healthy. The phone calls I received were caring and intended to bolster me, but also solicitous of information. People wanted to know concretely about the prevailing conditions. How was Marty doing, precisely? What was my state of mind? What was the schedule, in detail. Medical questions, to be sure, but also questions about what I was eating and where I was staying and what I did with myself all day. Phil, especially, barraged me with questions I could not answer. I began to feel an accusation in his voice I am sure he did not intend. I was quickly growing oppressed by those conversations and resentful of the obligation I was beginning to feel to reward every caller with a piece of my insides. Arline's calls were different. She could tell from my tone of voice all she needed to know. She would join me in a day or two. I needed her. Mom told me in every conversation how hard it was for her

179

to bear, how much it was wearing her down. Annoyed, I finally reminded her that it was Marty who would undergo the transplant.

Scolding myself for the petulant answer, I knew I had only myself to blame. From the time of the change in Marty's health until the present, I had assumed the role of his spokesman for the rest of our family. It was a proper role, I reasoned, because, outside of Vilunya, Leah and Aaron, I had the greatest contact with him. But there was also a certain amount of bravado in accepting that role. I would be in the center of the drama, hearing the expressions of concern for Marty and for me, sometimes deriving a ham actor's satisfaction from my role. And, indeed there were roles. With some people I would convey the full sense of the situation with all subtleties, not hiding anything. Others would get headlines, and for still others, like Mom, I would never share my forebodings and would deliberately withhold bad news. She made it clearly known that she wasn't strong enough, nor did she prefer to hear the step by step news of Marty's decline, from relative health to mortal illness.

People were justified, then, in calling on me to bring them up to date. The annoyance I now felt, the added burden of having to play press secretary after a day at the hospital, was merely part of the territory I had carved out. It would have to change. I didn't think I had the strength to do much more than participate in the transplant and attend to Marty daily, that is, to let him see me, his mirror, in a healthy condition.

To make that transition I realized the necessity of adopting a better, more healthful daily routine. While at the hospital I would be in the grip of Marty's schedule. But I determined that whenever I had a block of time during the day I would put it to constructive use and, in the evening, when I left the hospital I would read rather than molder in front of the accursed television. Planning my free time gave a certain pleasure: getting maps of the city and surrounds, walking through the Yale campus, exercising at a nearby health club, looking at some of the buildings in the vicinity designed by world famous architects, measuring my day, observing some of the world outside the hospital, diverting my obsessive thoughts of Marty.

Marty was lower the next morning. The chemotherapy was producing an immediate and strong reaction. He had puked up his breakfast and he was lying in his bed looking defensive, as if he was trying to find a position that would not further upset his stomach. He responded weakly to attempts at conversation and after a short time it became apparent that speaking was nausea-producing so we sat in silence. He seemed relieved when the nurse drew the curtain to help him in his very precise four times a day hygiene routine.

To remove any host for infection Marty had to use a powerful disinfectant to clean his ears, penis and anus. He had to swallow a foul-tasting substance to keep his digestive tract clean. It cleaned him so thoroughly that he told me his feces ceased to smell. When he defecated he used a portable potty set up in his room lined with a plastic bag. After he moved his bowels his feces were removed and weighed, another step in the careful monitoring he was subject to his entire stay in the hospital.

Barbara was Marty's nurse that morning. Although she had only recently begun to work in the transplant Unit she was regarded as a regular. After only a few days observation it was apparent that the Unit nurses were different from the other ward nurses. The obvious difference was in the ratio between nurses and patients. In the unit it was virtually one to one, in the general wards probably one to ten or fifteen. The Unit nurses did not face the variety of complaints of the general hospital population. They dealt exclusively with the problems of end stage leukemia and the terrible, but fairly repetitive difficulties caused by bone marrow transplant. The ones that I knew best during my stay at the hospital, Angela, Barbara and Hannah, were constant and authoritative in their ministrations. They brooked very little interference in their scheduled duties and in moments between organized chores they were always looking in on patients, just observing. The doctors, Rappeport and his assistant, Dr. Haroon Ahmad, in serious consultation with the nurses, frequently asked them questions, including their opinion of patients' conditions.

Hannah and Barbara were contrasts. Barbara, middle aged, small, dark haired with an unlined olive complexion, was a daughter of the Mediterranean. Energetic, she moved quickly and performed tasks with a flurry. She had a brooding expression much of the time. When she smiled it was a reward.

Hannah, was large, wide, fair, beyond middle age. Her expression seldom varied, giving her the aspect of a stern authoritarian, an impression heightened by the trace of the native Danish still in her speech. She had been on the unit quite a while. She had seen many patients come and go, some to cure and some to death. Her Scandinavian rectitude would not allow her to speculate or give unrealistic encouragement to the family of patients, something that, whether we asked for it openly or not, we all wanted. She did her job briskly and well.

Barbara was speaking to Marty through the plastic wall, asking him banal questions in a uncharacteristically stentorian voice. I heard her from the other room. A minute or two later, as she was walked past me, I asked her what that was all about. She told me she was testing Marty for confusion or disorientation, a possible side effect of Ara-C. She concluded that he was slightly displaying some of those symptoms, not in sufficient strength to be concerned about yet.

Vilunya was staying with Randy and Rita who had bought a house looking out on Long Island Sound. They were giving a barbecue that night to which I was invited and somewhat reluctantly agreed to come. When I arrived the party was in full progress. The house was ablaze with light, people circulating happily, drinks in hand. I was greeted warmly by both Rita and Randy and introduced immediately to the several knots of people close by. I was glad I had not refused the invitation. It was a much better choice than returning to my empty room, where I would be drawn into brooding thoughts. The house was full of life, of gayety. Most of the people there seemed to be engaged in some aspect of medical practice. Some were colleagues of Randy's, from his hospital, others, friends of Rita's, who was a health care consultant.

Everyone was excited. Whether the subject was the new health care plan being worked on by the Clinton administration, now less than eight months in office, or sailing in the sound, or a trip to the Galapagos being planned by a husband and wife concerned with environmental and tropical medicine, or the usual, the mundane; work and family, everyone was animated, gesticulating as they spoke, laughing without restraint. I circulated, I ate and drank and watched and listened with relish. It had been a long time since I had done this. The crowd rearranged itself slightly and I sighted Vilunya across the room in a small group. Her head was thrown back in laughter, her eyes shining with delight. Someone near me said, with shocked surprise, "Her husband is having a bone marrow transplant?"

Marty's image fell on me like a weight. If he was still awake lying in his hospital bed he was listening only to the muted sounds of the night shift nurses as they performed their duties quietly. Physically unable to enjoy any of things animating the people at the party even if he were here, Marty would have to lay quietly in his bed for yet more weeks, isolated from the pleasures I was now experiencing, enduring great suffering until he knew whether he had a chance to survive.

I bring him into the large, festive, noisy, room. Healthy and robust looking, perhaps from sailing in the sound for the day with Randy and Rita, I follow him with my eyes as he snakes his way through the mob, commenting to those he recognizes, excusing himself to others with his shy smile, arriving at a table of drinks and finger food. He peruses the offerings, making a serious, frowning, appraisal of the array of food, finally selecting a mouthful or two from several plates. Sated for the moment, he reads the labels of the open wine bottles, pours himself a glass and tastes it. From the barely perceptible narrowing of his eyes I conclude that for his next glass he will choose another wine. The glass held by the stem, his other hand in his pocket, he turns to assay the room. Like a slow motion broken field runner he makes his way into the thick of the milling crowd. A head flies up ten feet ahead and a voice cries out, "Hey Marty, come here." Handshakes, a partial embrace and introductions to two people he was to meet for the first time. Brought into the group, brief background notes exchanged, a summary of the topic they were discussing is given. He is asked his opinion. He counters with a delicately put question. He seeks to refine the answer with another question. His eyes narrow and he cocks his head slightly. He is adversarial to the point of view. Not that he disagrees entirely with what is said. He has a slightly different take, one that results in a conclusion a few crucial degrees from the present consensus. He introduces his belief, surrounds it with information not yet offered and, in no time, causes a mixture of confusion and admiration in his listeners. He looks over at me and flashes a jubilant, ironic, stained toothed smile.

Several days later I drove to New York to pick up Arline, our youngest daughter, Sharon, who was in New York for several weeks and my first cousin Selma, who lives there. How good it was to see Arline and know that I would have her close to me during the difficult time soon to come; to be able to talk to someone other than my fellow vigil keepers.

Selma, a life-long New Yorker, is both street hard and an intellectual. She has worked as an editor for many years, and reporter specializing in medical subjects. She can wither an opponent with a phrase and, minutes later, choke with laughter over some silly, often repeated bit of family lore. Selma, Phil's age, was raised in Brooklyn, not far from us. She is like a younger sister to Marty and me.

Sharon and her husband Keith are actors and mimists. They have traveled to several continents performing their show, part mime and part physical theater. They were in New York filming a children's mime video they had created, a venture fraught with anxiety for them both. Sharon is dark, bird-slight and fragile looking. Actually much tougher than her appearance, she is also very emotional. I was worried that Sharon might burst into tears and drag down our artificially elevated spirits. She had to return to New York the following day.

On the way to New Haven Arline was full of tales of the newly arrived Asa, answering the few questions left after the exquisite detail of her narration. Sharon explained the workings of putting together a video and Selma, from her experience, held forth animatedly about medical matters. We laughed a lot and scarcely talked of Marty.

We found Marty lively, rosy-cheeked and full of cheer as we all crowded into the space near his plastic curtain. He had been given a blood transfusion that afternoon. It produced an exaggeratedly high color to his face, a sick ruddiness. It raised his spirits and energy markedly. The contrast, between the low state he was in before the transfusion and the high, animated state after, was unsettling.

Arline, melting at the sight of Marty, immediately put her hands into the plastic gauntlets so that she could hold his hands in greeting. Sharon, visibly upset at the sight of Marty in isolation, approached him tentatively, carefully controlling her reaction. We visited a while, self consciously repeating much of the same discussion we had had in the car earlier. I removed myself to a chair in the corridor watching from behind, the group engulfing Marty, now swollen by Vilunya, Leah and her boy friend, newly arrived from California, and listened to the crescendo of their voices.

Almost without fail, people who were visiting Marty for the first time would play the role, according to their individual understanding of it, of minister to him. Some would be relentlessly cheery, prattling vacuously of things nobody cared about, anxiously ticking off the minutes of the visit. Others, lowering their voices becoming graver and more confiding, would try to impart to Marty their deep feeling, as if that expression could be left as a talisman to be clutched in their absence, its restorative powers continuing to work. Some would, by their voice and actions, try to dismiss the leukemia, the transplant, relegate it to a place of no importance. With loud, bluff, voice, they would talk of current events, Central American politics, weather, sailing, sports, as if to say that it was agreed that Marty was separated from these things only temporarily, soon to join these daily interests as the annoyance of the transplant was quickly eliminated. This response called to mind Carlos Castaneda, those many years ago, when he dismissed the notion of leukemia as something so fleeting that one need not be concerned with it, only to disappear without a word.

Everyone who visited Marty could see how dangerous his condition was. It was startlingly apparent just by looking at him in his bed, weakened by the disease and the therapies, surrounded by the extensive medical paraphernalia, that his life was in the balance. Despite the preparation they thought they had made to compose themselves, it took a while for visitors to adjust to the grim reality of Marty's situation. One visit was not enough.

Vilunya, Leah and I were the most frequent visitors. For the month I was in New Haven I was at the hospital every day, except for a two day respite. Though it was Marty imprisoned in his bed, I am sure that at times, they, like I, felt trapped by the circumstances. There were times when I presented myself to Marty just like a first time visitor, acting a role and wishing I were somewhere else.

I could tell without seeing him, from the raucous voices pouring out into the corridor, that Marty was enjoying the visit. Even though he was hidden from me by his visitors, the periodic silence from our side of the plastic wall followed by laughter, attested to Marty's jocular participation. He was hidden from me but I knew he was there. I could feel him. I was aware of him. In subsequent days, though, I would feel him drift away. How far and whether he would return, I would fearfully wonder about.

It is a bitter, windy March day, a day of dangerous possibilities. Heavy, dark clouds are blowing swiftly across the sky. We are seven years old, playing in the small back yard of our apartment building on Union Street. It is covered in dusty, frost-heaved concrete except for a patch of dirt, weeds and construction debris; broken bricks, aged scrap lumber with nails still attached, an attractive environment for Marty and me to graze in and select the props for our games. A window from our apartment, high up in the building, looks out over the yard from which our mother looks at us from time to time. A high board fence is the boundary between the yard and the garages attached to the single family houses that front on the next street. The garages, whose pointed, shingled roofs rose in orderly attention, seem as strange to us as minarets. They belong to people who possess cars and live in single family houses, characteristics outside of the experience of our family. The next street is a terrain we do not explore. Marty and I play in the lee of the fence as the wind swirls around us.

The game is our usual: a wild imaginary flight rescripted every few minutes and acted with all our little boys' zeal. The language between us is a grunted imperative—"you be the pirate, I'll be the captain of the navy ship." "Okay, then I'll be the native, you be the sailor." The real language is in the gestures of the hand, and body, the facial grimaces. The game is too important to dwell on the fine points. We work those out in performance, or if we can't, and our positions become intractable, we resort to the logic of fists and knees and elbows. Today the game is at its highest moment, each part fitting seamlessly into the other. Neither one covets the other's role. Each one, with high drama, wins glory and victory and acclaim in his persona. Our attention to the game is complete.

Suddenly, a groaning, a fast, violent creaking and then the crack that sounds like a gunshot, and the fence, six feet high, falls over on Marty in a slow motion, a malevolent undulation. An octopus, a manta ray, a foul giant spider, enfolds Marty in its deadly grip and prepares to devour him in its protected lair. He is trapped under the fence. I watch without moving. Marty, there a minute ago, is gone.

I run to the fence. I hear his muffled cries for help, but I can't see him. He is gone, only his cries, growing successively weaker, remain. He will never again appear. I am alone. I try to lift the fence. It is impossible. I scream wildly, with all the strength and volume possible from my little frame, my mouth and lungs stinging from the icy air.

Something fortuitous guides Mrs. Feldman's gaze at that moment to the fence. Her window is perhaps ten feet above the concrete surface below. Elderly Mrs. Feldman, in her house dress and slippers, flings her window open and leaps to the ground, her gray hair flying wildly. I watch as she flies to the fence, her feet not seeming to touch the ground, and with one hand raises the fence a foot or so and with the other reaches under and grabs Marty, drags him out and drops the fence. She is not aware that she has broken her ankle until later. Marty is hurt, bruised, but able to walk.

I can't remember what happened immediately after the rescue—what Marty's reaction is, what our mother's reaction is, whether she smacks both of us in an outburst of relief at not losing Marty and to assuage her guilt at not supervising us properly or whether she smacks me for not preventing the near tragedy or just envelops Marty in her bosom, grateful at his escape from disaster. I remember nothing further of Mrs. Feldman, although I will recall her when I see her husband, a slight, stooped, elderly man, walking to the subway with a shuffling, palsied gait, wearing a business suit and carrying a diplomat's briefcase. We thought he had a good job, a desk job, until we were older and found out that he was a messenger on Wall Street and he carried his lunch in his briefcase. Nothing remains in memory except the awful, never to be forgotten, events surrounding the fence falling on Marty. Beyond that, I can only remember the feeling in my stomach, of a dead, aching, of the air being sucked out of me. I still love the memory of Mrs. Feldman, who saved Marty, who saved us both.

The crowd outside of the plastic curtain began to separate and I joined the visitors to add my good-byes. Sharon and Marty were smiling sweetly at each other, each not wanting the other to be distressed. Sharon was sobered, but she held her tears. Marty was still taking care of those visitors who he felt were overreacting to the sight of him: acting stronger than he felt, understating the severity of his state, being optimistic about his prognosis. We left the hospital and split into two groups—Vilunya and her contingent to Rita and Randy's house in Branford and Arline, Selma, Sharon and I to a local Italian restaurant.

Marty was out for the first total body radiation (TBI) when we arrived Monday morning, August 9, 1993, three days before the transplant. While we waited for him to return, I witnessed the discharge of Pon. Today was the day he would leave behind the plastic walled room and the hospital and reenter a world of freedom and danger. I saw him, slouched in his wheelchair as he went by me, barely strong enough to return the expressions of encouragement offered by everyone on the unit at that moment, both staff and visitors. When I had seen him a couple of days before, he looked very sick. Now, leaving the hospital, he didn't seem much healthier. Dr. Smith told me they used to have a party every time a patient was discharged. They no longer do it because discharge is so commonplace. How encouraging it was to hear that. It boded well for Marty.

Marty returned in good spirits with a high color. He told us that they had toasted him lightly on both sides. He was not throwing up and the headache that had plagued him for a day or two was gone. For today and tomorrow he would have the radiation twice a day and would start on Cyclophosphamide (Cytoxan), the last of the high dose chemotherapy. When those therapies were fully administered he would have about a day and a half to wait to receive the new marrow. The chemicals were a systemic poison to kill the leukemic cells that still existed and the radiation would finish off all of Marty's marrow. That was the theory. Then, free of cancer the new healthy marrow will colonize in his body and start producing healthy cells and he'll be cured. He was not yet feeling the full effects of the chemotherapy and the radiation. The next few days would be rough.

Before and after each total body radiation he has to be washed thoroughly to enable him to return to his sterile environment as free of foreign agents as possible, and, I suppose, to rid the skin of any lingering effect of the radiation. During the TBI, he has to hold a pose for 15 or 20 minutes on each side. Although he experiences no pain during the radiation, holding the position tires him. I had read about total body radiation treatments of not many years ago when the patient was placed in a coffin-like box and bags of rice were wedged between the patient and the sides of the box. The radiation treatment, absolutely necessary before the transplant, renders the patient sterile. It did not matter in Marty's case, because he has two grown children. It had an awful sound to me though, being bombarded with rays that removed an important aspect of manhood. Marty was not particularly disturbed by what I perceived to be a loss, even if a symbolic one. It took me a while to realize how different our vantage points were.

I was still rooted in daily life. The subtle, accretive, proofs of the diminution of powers and abilities that I experienced were overwhelmed by vanities which argued that I was young and strong and would remain so forever. Marty was beyond that. Nothing much mattered to him beyond staying alive. There was almost no loss he would not have accepted to remain alive. He was realistic in the way that only one who has looked into the pit can be. Not being able to have more children was academic, theoretic. Staying alive, with hair, without hair, damaged, diminished, but with the ability to work, to read, to enjoy those aspects of life still available to him, that was real. The medical staff was always admonishing Marty to be a fighter against his disease. They would put it in a way that I found somewhat condescending. "We don't want quitters around here. We want fighters. You have to help us lick this thing."

Marty once asked me, with strong annoyance, what they meant by that exhortation. I looked at him in amazement. I could not imagine anyone who considered his situation with greater singularity than Marty. Other aspects of his life, those of lesser importance than survival, were being abandoned. His concentration was fixed on what his body was going through. His expression, at times, intense and inward, withdrawing from the activities on the other side of the curtain, banishing the extraneous, reminded me of a preacher about to do battle with the devil.

Sterility was not a problem for Marty. Ray, in the next room, though, was 28 years old. I learned that he and his wife, who was then pregnant, had one child. I speculated that she became pregnant in anticipation of the transplant. A practical, sad, decision. Day after day she came, moving slowly, her step seeking counterbalance for her big belly, her clean, sweetly stoic face revealing nothing. She would smile a murmured greeting to me, and later, when we became accustomed to the sight of each other and had exchanged more extensive greetings, we would ask each other tentative questions, about her husband and Marty. It always touched me, watching her struggling clumsily to mount the high stool at the plastic wall to begin a visit with her husband, her awkward movements the deliberate defense of her unborn child even as she looked upon the father her child might never see.

Our gang was getting unwieldy. Rather than all eight of us, as we had grown to, visiting with Marty all at once, we broke into smaller groups. Some remained in the unit, others wandered away. Sharon and Selma were soon returning to New York.

I was beginning to feel oppressed by the non-stop visiting, the endless discussions, the intricate planning about where and what to eat. Irrelevant to the transplant, they distracted me from thinking and worrying about what would happen in three days.

We milled about the unit before disbursing. I talked with Dr. Ahmad. He told me, with a certain relish, that the harvesting always gives him a good workout. He said it improves the carpentry muscles. His comment made me feel like a piece of gym equipment.

The next morning I arrived alone after Marty had finished the radiation and was waiting for his bath. We talked about a book he had given me to read. A colleague of his had written what the dust jacket described as an anthropological account of his fatal illness, a spinal tumor. I couldn't tell why it should be considered anthropology, except that it seemed to be an unsparing account, revealing painful, often uncomplimentary descriptions of him. I liked the book, The Body Silent, by Robert Murphy. As the narrative advanced, the disease progressed, his pain increased and the writing grew better. I concluded that as his time grew shorter he was freed from the constraints of academic writing. He knew he would not be around to hear the criticisms of colleagues who would complain that he had strayed from the traditional method of presenting a study.

The phone in Marty's room rang while we were talking. It was Mom. I gathered from Marty's expression and his end of the conversation, that Mom was worried, needy, teary. Marty's responses were strong and upbeat. He advised her with a confidential surety, that everything would be all right. He had to almost shout into the phone. Mom could not get used to her "*fahkokte*" hearing aid. Marty and I smiled at each other, a smile that acknowledged without words a scene that we recalled from our youth.

189

Mom's sister and brother-in-law, Leda and Jack Victor, moved to Flushing from Brooklyn in the late forties. They bought a semi-detached house, my uncle Jack told me much later, for $7,000. Marty and I hated to make the journey from Brooklyn. It was always on a Sunday, robbing us of a whole day, normally reserved for playing basketball. The drive was interminable, even after we began making the trip in Dad's 1939 Nash Ambassador. The only, occasional compensations were seeing our cousins, Norman and Ed, with whom we weren't always on good terms, and playing with Fluffy, their old dog.

After the meal, in which prodigious quantities of food were consumed, Dad and Uncle Jack would go into the living room and smoke cigarettes while they talked of politics and the stock market, in the penumbra of the glowing artificial fireplace. Mom and aunt Leda sat at the now cleared dining room table and talked to each other in Russian and Yiddish. The kids would lie around, agitating for the adults to finish their conversations so we could go home.

Shifra and Mendel, our grandparents," zaide" and "bubbe", lived with the Victors then because, according to the custom, the elders lived with the daughter who had the best accommodations. Mendel was still active, assisting somewhat in the running of the household. He walked the dog, cleared the table, and occasionally washed the dishes. Always clean shaven, he wore a tie every day. He never failed to join us for family dinners, which he ate with a relish that was revealed in his face. He was transported by food. Ceremoniously, he would ladle the steaming soup into his mouth, pausing after every three or four spoonsful to bite off a piece of the dark bread he held at the ready. He seemed to be preoccupied with the food he was consuming, considering its qualities critically. His eyebrows would raise and lower, his shoulders shrug, his bread hand conducting a mimed autodialog. Was the soup hot enough? Was it seasoned satisfactorily? It never mattered. He invariably finished every morsel in his bowl or plate, lifted his face to display a radiant smile to his dining companions. Too subtle for us kids, his daughters knew precisely whether his expression meant that he was completely satisfied and would eat no more, could be persuaded to another helping or was actively soliciting more. They were never wrong and he was always obliging.

Shifra, on the other hand, lived like an invalid, dwelling mostly in her room, surrounded by her scents and potions. Sometimes she remained in her room during the entire visit. Before the visit could be rightfully concluded, however, Shifra had to bid us all a tearful farewell, complete with prayers for a peaceful world and a blessing on her grandchildren.

One winter evening the blessings and the prayers would not end. In Yiddish and the occasional Russian, and sporadically a word or two she thought was English, but which was unintelligible to us, she exhorted each of us, individually, to grow up and become prosperous and to insure our perpetual tranquillity, prayed that there be no war. The specter of war, rendered more real to her by the uttering of it, so troubled her that she repeated the blessings and prayers over again, while lavishing minty kisses on us. Dad was standing near the door dressed for the outdoors; overcoat, hat, gloves and scarf. After perhaps twenty minutes, there seemed to be no end in sight.

"You should grow up strong and be a doctor, an engineer. There shouldn't be a war." Each time she intoned the word war it pushed her further into a panicked, tearful, state that seemed to require her to say it yet again.

Dad was impatiently taking his hat off, smoothing his hair, reblocking his hat, putting it on again. Finally, with an audible exhalation, he snapped the brim of his hat down, snugging it against his brow, strode across the room quickly, and took both of Shifra's hands in his own. "Ma, Ma, there won't be a war." "No?" she said and fixed her rheumy eyes on his, seeking proof of the sincerity of his assertion. All action momentarily froze in the room as Shifra divined the true meaning of his words. Then, with a slight, tension relieving laugh, she said, "Very good. Let there not be a war." Her eyes dried instantly and she released whichever of us she was clutching. The visit ended seconds later as we flew out the door into the winter night amidst muffled farewells.

I sought the comfort of a routine. I was becoming frayed, annoyed or nervous over usual, daily, abundant inconveniences over which I had no control and which I would not have noticed in other circumstances. Arline calmed me somewhat. Together we did things unconnected to the transplant. We strolled around New Haven, went through the Kahn-designed British Art Museum, sampled the deservedly famous New Haven pizza.

I began to read William Kennedy's cycle of books, all set in Albany, New York. I had no sympathy at first for Kennedy's poor Irish characters. I had known very few people like them and had always heard them depicted as drunkards, wife beaters and slackers. I pictured them like the hospital laundry workers across Crown Street during our early teens: lank, stooped men, with gaunt, ill-shaved, colorless faces, in overcoats too big for them, snot icicles hanging from their noses in winter, who chased us off the large, steep lawn, flanked by the driveways leading to the main building, screaming "kike" and "sheeny" after us as we nimbly retreated, taunting them over our shoulders. We realized they were harmless when we would see them occasionally in Lee's candy store, shyly asking permission to saucer their coffee.

Kennedy brings us patiently and skillfully into the doleful lives of the inhabitants of a cold and grimy land. People who struggle to accommodate to ancient grievances too painful to forget, they toil away drearily, seeking some respite from the desolation in their lives. Conditioned by their early church instruction, they pine for, but learn not to expect, redemption. They are neither noble nor attractive. Most of the time they are not even interesting, but they bear their burden with a certain courage and without railing against their fate. They are unsettlingly real. Their failures are familiar to all of us, their hopes perhaps more modest.

Kennedy's writing complemented the gray and depressed mood I was struggling against. Somehow Marty was in those pages, living his hard life, grinding out one day after another, silently bearing his burden. Lying in his bed and waiting for the pain of the chemotherapy and radiation to wash over him, he began to disengage from what had always interested him. He virtually stopped reading and did not work at all on the book he was writing on El Salvador. He barely watched television except, it appeared, as a soporific. He listened much more than he spoke to visitors. At times his eyes lacked focus, making his withdrawal complete at that moment. He would look at a poster he had hung on the wall just outside his room that he could see through the open doorway, showing a wizened pair of peasants, dressed in country clothes, staring through brown, wrinkled, expressionless faces and captioned, ***STAYING ALIVE IN EL SALVADOR***. That's what Marty was doing—staying alive, using all his strength, physical and psychic, all his concentration, all his will. He had no strength for anything or anyone else. At first I thought he was slipping away from us, yielding to what his mind concluded was the inevitable, taking up permanent residence in that other land. Then it became apparent that his immediate condition bore more heavily than any other factor on his ability and desire to respond. His hearing was deteriorating, we would find out later.

Marty was feeling rotten the next morning. He was throwing up and had a raging diarrhea. Today he would have the last of the radiation treatments and tomorrow would be the transplant. He was afraid that, swathed in surgical dress on the way to the therapy, he would soil himself, or when he had to remain motionless he would be seized with convulsive retching and spoil the radiation. Or, worst of all, if his bowels let loose during the radiation he would have to lay in his own mess. Instead, happily, he fell asleep peacefully listening to Glenn Gould playing the Goldberg variations.

Mom called while he was being bathed after the radiation. Marty's voice grew animated, confident, assuring and calming her.

Mom could not wait to fish. She talked about it like a child during the drive to Greer. At 8,500 feet, I was slightly apprehensive as to how she and Dad, who had had a pacemaker installed recently, would tolerate the thin air. I settled her on the bank of a lake, swaddled in a down jacket, baited her hook and cast her line out. I carefully explained to her how to tell if she had a bite by watching the action of the bobber on the surface. Not given to thoughtful concentration, she surprised me by the intensity with which she approached this new experience. At the ready, almost in a crouch, she watched the bobber like an Eskimo poised over a hole in the ice, harpoon in hand, waiting for a seal to surface. Several times the bobber went under, the bait having been attacked from below. She impatiently bade me rebait her hook and cast out her line. Almost immediately the bobber went under and from the bent rod tip she could feel the fish she had hooked. I stood beside her, telling her how to bring the fish in. When at last it was thrashing on the ground at her feet, she looked at it with the appreciation of a climber having reached a summit. We repeated the process several more times, eating the result for dinner that night.

The next day I went with Dad to a nearby lake where we rented a boat. He carried a two-day-old newspaper and stood watching me with silent appreciation of my competence as I attached the battery and made the boat ready to launch. He asked questions about everything: birds, trees, clouds, water temperature, species of trout, the electric motor. Most answers he accepted with the pleasure of having acquired new knowledge. Some he doubted, without information to offer in rebuttal, when the response did not comport with his own experience, or perhaps it was just an instinctive distrust of his son's offering.

We were to do a little more serious fishing, I thought. I cruised the small lake slowly, trolling a nymph that had served me well in the past. I hoped to display my skill by picking up a fish or two and show Dad that it was possible for him to catch fish too. Nothing, not a bump. I anchored fifty feet or so from the small earthen dam and spillway, in the lee of a thick stand of trees, a beautiful, sheltered spot, ideal for quiet, restful fishing or, should the mood strike us, conversation. The alpine lake lay like a pearl at the foot of the surrounding steeply rising mountains, clothed in the healthy green of Ponderosa pine. Beyond the timber line, where the climate could not support the growth of trees, could be seen rocky outcroppings, mountain meadows, and the year round snow mantle of Mount Baldy, at 11,000 feet.

I rigged his line the same way I had Mom's, and began to show him how to cast. He took the rod from me before I had finished instructing him and, on his first cast, snarled the line. Patiently, I untangled the line, told him what he had done wrong and cast it out for him. On my first cast I had a small strike. As always happens at that moment I felt the current flow through me, heightening my concentration, filling me with a joyful tension. He was there, waiting for my next cast. With the right presentation, the fly in the proper place, the line skillfully manipulated on the retrieve, I'd have him.

"What's wrong with this reel? Every time I throw out the line it tangles," Dad, who was deaf, said, in a voice louder than he realized. I waved for him to pipe down, fearful that the sound would spook the fish. He stopped talking and began making a sound he thought was whistling, a loud, unmelodic hissing through his teeth. He was clearly not enjoying the fishing or even being out in a boat with me. I determinedly made a few more casts to no avail. Dad swished the tip of his rod through the water, further snarling the line. Clearly, the fishing was over. I reeled my line in, calmed myself and looked at Dad.

His whistling had become a series of low rhythmic exhalations, pounding out the beat of a Russian song, familiar to me since childhood. Absently making figures in the water with the rod tip, he looked out past me, across the lake, beyond the trees, to the mountains, through the trees and mountains, thinking, dreaming, lost somewhere, seeing his life cracked open, ambushed by a deeply imbedded thought, looking through the space and time of his life, seeing everything, seeing nothing. He remained like that for several minutes.

"If I had bought RCA stock in 1930 I would have made enough money to have brought my brothers and sisters to this country and they would not have perished." It was a clear, crisp, fluently delivered sentence. He looked directly at me. I don't know what he saw.

I had in mind that Marty needed a mental boost; that his sinking into despondency would hurt his chances for engrafting, that my marrow would be bogged down in gloom and darkness. He needed to feel encouraged, optimistic, loved, I reasoned, in order for his body to enthusiastically welcome my marrow, to cheer it on, to welcome it and escort it through well-lit tunnels and caverns in his body to the comfortable niches and nests where conditions would be perfect to set about the business of colonizing. I wrote him a letter, rewritten several times over a period of days, which

I envisioned being handed to him as my marrow was being infused into him. It was corny, or to be more elevated, more revelatory of my heart, than I could have spoken it directly to Marty.

The letter became magnified in my thoughts until it took the significance of a plan, an essential part of the therapeutic strategy whereby Marty would successfully engraft. So it was with a jolt that I realized that everything that went into Marty's room had to be sterilized. Today, in a matter of hours, the bag of whitish sludge would be delivered to Marty's and I was now uncertain if the letter could be introduced into his room. I stopped in to see Marty before I checked in to a different part of the hospital to begin my part in the transplant.

Fortunately, Rappeport was there. I told him about the letter, explained that I wanted Marty to be able to read it while he was being infused. With no fuss, Rappeport took it from me and said he would make an exception this once. I worried slightly that I would be introducing germs into his room, especially at this vulnerable moment for him, but I hoped, I believed, it would do more good than harm.

The part of the hospital I was installed in, a floor or two higher and in a different wing, was brighter and cheerier than the part Marty was in. The pastel colors and the almost eye hurting illumination buoyed me somewhat. It seemed an atmosphere in which germs could not avoid detection, in which infection was forbidden. I wished Marty was here, closer to me. I was grateful for the private room, sparing me from having to visit and make small talk with a stranger.

Changed into the hospital attire, I sat in the bed and received the people who would prepare me for the procedure. First, the blood letter, who filled a couple of vials. Then the anesthetist, younger than my son, who explained the options; to be awake but feel no pain or to be knocked out. I elected to be knocked out. A young intern tried to install an I.V. in my arm. After two tries he quit. A nurse took over. She had her two tries. My veins are very prominent, so it was hard for me to understand why they were having so much difficulty. It was explained to me that my veins were rolling. Bad veins, naughty veins. Sit still for the nice people. Don't give them a hard time. A grossly overweight, loud-voiced nurse with wild orange hair barreled into the room and immediately made me feel comfortable that she was the ward expert in I.V. setting. She got it in on the second try, leaving me with five black and blue marks. Nothing to do now but wait.

I would have preferred waiting alone, attempting to bring myself into a state of calm, but the room filled up with well wishers. A tentative kiss, a careful hug, a good luck wish from a shy, averted eye from across the room. Leah, Aaron, Vilunya were there as was Ellen, a friend from New York, up for the day to keep Arline company while I was "out." Vilunya presented me with a book depicting a type of Mexican handicraft called Milagros (miracles). She nervously held forth on the meaning of those miracles until every one in the room became edgy and finally, someone asked her to stop. It was time to go anyway. Everyone's good wishes trailed after the gurney as I was being wheeled out, flanked only by Arline and Ellen. The automatic doors to the holding area of the operating rooms slammed behind us and I was pushed into a corner to wait. Arline looked drawn and fearful. She was successfully controlling her tears. I said things to soothe and calm her. The game that I had seen played so many times recently was that the patient has to take care of those around him until he is no longer able and then the reverse must begin. I would have a few minutes of it. Marty had been doing it for years. I was approached by a surgical gowned man, gauze face mask hanging at his throat, one rubber gloved hand holding a syringe, the other lining up the end of the I.V. lumen. Checking the strap that held me in the gurney, he said, "I'm going to give you some stuff that will relax you and make you drowsy."

The constricting tension, the light buzz of electrical current that holds my skin and muscles in its grip, begins rapidly to melt. As the surface tension dissolves, it transforms from a unified effect, a blanket covering, to an infinite number of tiny weights that seeps beneath the skin, each weight attaching itself, one by one, onto every cell of the body, uniformly increasing the pull of gravity, drawing the will out of every separate part of the body, negating any thought, desire or impulse, to move. There it lays, that body, being observed by the last flicker of wakeful comprehension in a mind still vaguely connected to me. It has no weight, no arch to the small of the back, the foot exerting no leverage on the ankle, the hands not caring or noticing whether their palms were facing up or down. The body is light—oh, so light. The strap around the midsection securely holds it down, preventing it from floating toward the ceiling. The mind, a fraction of it still my mind, clean and airy as a cloud, welcomes every thought and sensation, exults without sound or motion or sign of awareness, in the precise, absolute, present. There is Arline, at that moment hovering above me, not bounded by the frame of the photograph on the wall of our bedroom in Phoenix, her arms embracing her folded legs, her strong hands forming the clasp, her face in three quarter profile, the angled sunlight casting a faint, powerful, sexy shadow in the hollow beneath her high cheekbone, her eyes regarding the future with optimism and courage, equally prepared for either struggle or love. "Feeling fine. Not worry. Everything all right."

The body is too heavy and dense to think of trying to move it. The mouth and throat are stuffed with cotton permeated with dried persimmon talcum powder. The head is feeling an unpleasant buzz, the brain too mangled to attempt thought. At the moment all that is possible is to try to make sense of the visual and auditory impressions. A department store, the floor space bordered by counters laden with chrome equipment, uniformed attendants, mostly women, operating the equipment with bang and crash. The overhead, undeflected light bearing down with an intensity that forces the eyes into defensive slits, presaging an ache in the head. The toe at the other end moves, observed humorously by the eye. A hand raises, drawn to within inches of the eyes, fingers wriggles with increasing speed. A tentative, gentle flexing of the calf muscles, a pelvic thrust against the leather strap. Then a stretch of the chest and shoulders, leveraged with upraised arms, several deep breaths, and finally, I am able to raise my head and look around.

A sturdily built nurse approached me, appraisingly. She put a hand on my chest, a gesture I appreciated. "You think you're strong enough to move over to this gurney by yourself?" I raised my upper body some inches, hinged at the strap. The truncated sentence formed by my brain never exited my mouth audibly. The sound I uttered was mush. With smacking noises, I unglued my mouth. "I think so." Then, slowly, with deliberation, looking directly at the nurse, to convince her of my return to mental and physical acuity, I said, "My body works better than my mouth." She smiled a tolerant smile, undid the strap and with encouraging grunts and a hand supporting my back, guided me onto the gurney that was to bear me back to my room.

Arline's face gradually came into focus in the corridor as they returned me to my room. She was rubbing her fingernail along her lip, a comforting habit, her face illuminated with relief when she saw me. She kissed me and stroked my face after I got into bed. I acknowledged her ministrations dumbly. Other friends were in the room, Barbara and Paul from New Hampshire. People asked me how I felt. I assured everyone that I felt all right. Fatigued, I mumbled how well I felt to no one in particular. Arline asked everyone to leave and I fell asleep immediately.

August 12, 1993
My Marty,

A long time ago, when we were cubs rolling around in our self-created den, when the experience of one was shared by the other, when the world considered us as one and we responded as one, we didn't need words between us to convey our thoughts or describe our moods. Now, after having lived apart almost three times as long as we lived together, we do. Not as many words as mere siblings perhaps, but after the long absence from each other in time and distance and the different lives we have lived, I am drawn - obliged - to speak to you clearly, as an adult.

Since your illness worsened two years ago or so and, more particularly, since we spoke of death in Telluride last year, I have felt and imagined the unbearable pain of being without you. It is the feeling of having some integral part of me physically torn out of me, something living in me, but not entirely mine.

I would survive your death as you would survive mine. But something that I could not easily explain or describe to anyone else but you would be finished for me, would be stilled forever; that part of me that we had in common as children, that part that never fully separated from each other. I have felt closer to that secret part of us this last year or so than I have since we were children.

Although at times I didn't feel it was a good thing to be twins, I feel favored by fate to be twins with you now. Being able to exchange a part of our body is sweetly appropriate. But that is the mechanical part. The rest of what I give you comes from that secret place we share, from a place deeper than my heart. That magma of feeling, of love for you, is with you. Feel it in your brain, in your gut. It will draw you. It will pull you, to me, to your family and friends, to your productive life, to health. Think of it, dear Marty, when things get bad. Focus on it. Use it. Let it pull you back to us.

Come back to us all soon and come back to your
Sauly

I had dreamt of being there, seeing the moment of the transfer of marrow from the plastic bag to Marty, but had I thought about it realistically I would have realized that it was impossible. As soon as the marrow was extracted and processed it was given to Marty. Fresh from the cow. I was still semi-conscious while the infusion was occurring. I was told that those present at the actual moment the marrow was entering his body were sobbing watching Marty read my letter. The tears were the flood of hope. All the dammed worry and fear was being released as if the successful conclusion was very near. Just a matter of the marrow colonizing, and the counts, particularly the white blood cells, restoring themselves. A matter of a few weeks to cure.

Later that day, maybe six o'clock in the evening, I called the Unit and asked for someone to take me over to see Marty. Barbara, from the Unit, appeared shortly, to appraise my condition. Within seconds she vetoed the plan. "You're in no condition to go anywhere." That was that. She was right. I fell into a deep sleep as soon as she left my room.

When I awoke several hours later, I tried a different tactic, not wanting my plan to be again vetoed. I asked one of the nurses on my wing to call for an orderly to transport me to the BMT unit. Without questioning, she did it. In a few minutes an elderly, light-skinned black man appeared at my door with a slip of paper, informing me that he was there to make the delivery. He was whistling what sounded like swing tunes of the forties. I arose, rocky and lurching, slightly dizzy. I struggled into a bathrobe, shivering. He never looked in my direction, distractedly continuing his whistling. The gurney poked into the room, perhaps three paces from the bed. The first full step I took produced a powerful dizzyness and, explosively, I threw up into a small sink. After thirty seconds or so, the spasms subsided and gripping the sink with one hand for balance, I washed my face with the other, laboriously mounted the gurney and off we went to the soft accompaniment of my tuneful chauffeur.

It was a long way to the Unit. At least, it felt that way. During the journey I could feel every bump and unevenness in the floor. The walls and ceiling glided by, changing in texture and illumination as we moved from the newer wing to the older one. The halls became narrower, the lighting more subdued, and in places, we plunged into a blackness that felt more like an entry into another, more problematic, world. The hospital was silent, the patients asleep or quiescent, all the maintenance employees gone until tomorrow and only a skeletal version of the medical staff remained. I was content to lie still on the gurney, letting my stomach settle and my mind clear, not overly eager to arrive.

Marty was sitting up in bed, fully awake. The orderly navigated the gurney close to the plastic curtain. He did it artfully, silently, without bumping anything, and without a word, left on padded feet, his whistling diminuendo the only sign of his leave-taking. I raised myself to an upright position on the gurney, slowly, to ward off the dizziness and the nausea, my legs dangling, my head at about the same level as Marty's. We greeted each other in voices barely above a whisper. Marty regarded me carefully, inspecting me for signs of wear or stress.

"How are you feeling? Did it go okay? "

"It went well so far as I know. I would've come sooner but I'm a little groggy, I guess, from the anesthesia. How about you? Did the infusion go well? How long ago did you get it?"

"Early in the afternoon. You were probably still out. Did you elect to be conscious during the harvest or did you get a general?"

"A general. I wasn't aware of anything until it was over."

"Good."

I put my hands in the plastic gauntlets, inserting my fingers into the gloves. Marty took both my hands in his and we sat quietly, holding hands and looking at each other for several minutes without speaking. After a time he took my rubber glove-encased hand and held it to his face and head.

"I read your letter while the marrow was being infused. It meant everything to me. Things were very emotional around here, for me and everyone else. Thanks, thanks, for everything."

"You're welcome."

We spoke in husky, throat-clearing tones, grateful to return to silence. We sat quietly, observing whether any changes had been made in either one of us by the transfer of marrow. Hannah announced with a bustling noise that she was approaching. Careful not to embarrass us by looking either of us full in the face, she suggested that we consider the visit ended. The guttural remnants of her native tongue made the suggestion seem like a command, one we were both pleased to obey. It had been a long and draining day. The visit had accomplished its purpose. I saw Marty, touched him, and had proof that he was still alive. Marty mirrored that ritual behavior for the first time in the course of his illness. He looked at me in a familiar way. It was the same way I was accustomed to looking at him in recent years: critically, with a diagnostic eye, in an effort to determine his state of health and the degree of damage, if any. Now I was also weakened, perhaps damaged. I showed all the evidence of it, dressed in a hospital gown, sitting on the edge of a gurney, obviously unsteady, probably with a gray pallor, recovering from the anesthesia. Marty had to determine whether I was hurt or ill or suffering any untoward consequences of the bone marrow harvest. He looked at me, touched me, spoke to me and had the proof of his senses and intellect that I was still alive and probably none the worse for wear. Discreetly, Hanna didn't insist on speaking to me on the way back to my room. I lay on the gurney, sleep closing in on me as I pondered the gifts Marty and I had exchanged that day.

There were some unpleasant side effects of the marrow harvest. I had a shooting pain on one side of my pelvis and down the attached leg. The other one had a strange, sometimes painful sensation, something like a small firecracker going off from time to time in my thigh. In the middle of these two annoyances was a formidable black and blue mark radiating from my tailbone, a hemotoma as big as my hand. One of the doctors involved in the harvest, to whom I mentioned these symptoms, said to me, "Oh yeah, we must've nicked a nerve and a blood vessel or a vein." He didn't seem to be overly concerned about it, and so, for the time being, my fears were allayed. There were perhaps ten punctures, front and back, each the size of a large pinhead. I had to wear a dressing over them for a few days to prevent infection.

I slept sporadically that night, awaking many times. Arising in considerable pain in the morning, I faced a cheery procession of hospital staff introducing themselves to me. Andrea, Devon, Kerry, and at last, a young red-curled intern …Dr. Matt something. He and one of the nurses kept offering me morphine for the pain. I was reluctant to accept because I was still somewhat groggy from the anesthesia and I wanted to be sure of what I was feeling before I took any new drug. Arline and Ellen stayed with me, asking to do things for me. I was out of sorts, slightly depressed, I later concluded. Toward noon Ellen left for New York. Arline took her to the station and I slept.

Barbara and Paul came by. Paul bombarded me with jokes and witticisms. I wasn't in the mood for it, but I had no way to stop it. Paul was uncomfortable. A philosopher of religion, he is usually a serious man. I could see in his eyes he didn't like the way I looked and he was trying to cheer me, to enliven me. I could see how hard it was for him to decide the most appropriate way to behave but I couldn't instruct him at that moment. I must have done what I'd seen Marty do; retreat into a frozen silence.

The air grew heavy until Aaron entered the room wearing a blank expression, conveying concern beneath the mask, surveying the room. He approached me quickly and kissed me gently, his eyes full of feeling, and addressed me as Uncle Saul, a title I love. Aaron was a different young man now than he had been last December at Marty's splenectomy. He was content to observe, without demanding attention, helping when needed. It seemed almost as if he sensed the historical irony. He was the child Vilunya had become pregnant with after their newborn baby died. Although his birth went well, it was a nervous pregnancy. Both Marty and Vilunya were frightened that something would go wrong. In an abundance of caution, Vilunya stayed in bed for part of the time so as not to dislodge the fetus. Almost as soon as it was certain that he would survive, that he was strong and healthy, Marty was diagnosed with CLL. Aaron was the baby that Marty wasn't sure he would live to see grow up. Now Marty needed Aaron's help and he was quickly growing into the part.

The room began to fill with visitors and the mood lightened considerably. After a while we all decided to walk over to the unit and visit with Marty. We walked in a group, in a relaxed fashion, slowly as an accommodation to me, chattering lightheartedly. Everything seemed normal, usual, routine. A group composed of family and friends, strolling aimlessly, without a pressing schedule, confident that all was well. It was what I needed: a public acknowledgment that there was no imminent disaster. The moment of transplant had passed with no dramatic surprises. On to the next phase. Perhaps the most difficult and dangerous one of all, but for the time being I sank into the general air of contentment that Marty was still alive and so was I.

Our entourage arrived at the Unit to find Marty throwing up and coughing up the phlegmy mucosa his body was sloughing off. After his violent coughing and puking bout he looked up at the small crowd assembled at the plastic curtain with a red-faced smile, full of puckish drama, and although teary from the exertion, he was ready for the encounter with the mob of visitors. He was in quite a social mood. I greeted him briefly and withdrew to a chair while the others visited with him. Loud voices knifed the air of the Unit as his visitors vied for his attention and choruses of laughter responded to Marty's humor. The room seemed to be full of smiles and lightened hearts. Aaron circulated through the group, snapping pictures constantly, recording everyone's participation.

I was annoyed by the levity outside Marty's room. It seemed to me that the high spirits were the group's acknowledgment that everything would be all right, that the transplant was a success and Marty's recovery a certainty. It seemed a display of hubris to me, a premature celebration. We trouped back to my room, from where everyone departed and left me alone with my gloomy thoughts.

Later, after dinner, I went back to the Unit to watch a Boston Red Sox game with Marty. I sat on a high stool, uncomfortably watching the game from outside the plastic curtain. The game didn't interest me and it was difficult to see well through the plastic, but I sat to keep Marty company. It was strangely amusing to me that Marty was a genuine sports fan. Our visit was interrupted by his periodic bursts of coughing, retching and vomiting. Each succeeding bout left him more fatigued, until he finally dozed off. I wandered off to the other room where I encountered Rappeport reading a patient's chart, holding the pages down with his elbows while raining crumbs upon it from the ossified Danish he was eating, which he was vainly trying to soften with the stale coffee he was absentmindedly drinking.

It was well after nine o'clock and Rappeport had been in the hospital since early that morning. Apparently, that was a usual day for him. Tonight, instead of his usual approachable demeanor the Rapster looked drained. The drooping flesh on his longish face had a yellowish cast. His eyes were vacant. He looked like his body was begging for bed, but some problems unsolved, some answer eluding him was keeping him here.

He willingly interrupted his unsavory snack to chat with me for a while. He held forth with some heat about the ills of the health care system. His principal complaint was that it was burdened with bureaucracy, his particular gripe related to what he considered the top heavy administrative apparatus that interfered with medical decisions and drew money away from patient services. Much of his argument, I thought, derived from his frustration at not being able to cure everyone who came under his care. Frightened by the thought that he might be considering Marty's case bleak, I asked him guardedly, but without preface, how Marty was doing. His face grew taut and the focus immediately came back in his eyes. He told me it was too soon to be making predictions but that he was hopeful that there would be a good outcome. His canned comment, delivered without affect, indicated the conversation was over. He left a moment later. I was sorry I had returned him to the subject he could not discuss with me. I looked in on Marty. He was sleeping restlessly, snoring arhythmically. I left the Unit.

Chilled and weary and somewhat downcast, drawing my robe closer around me, I trudged what now loomed as a great distance toward my room across the sleeping hospital. Fatigue was overtaking me, and with that fatigue a fear that I wouldn't have the strength to make it back to my room. The atmosphere of the long, desolate corridors was threatening. Strange noises came from unseen quarters: regretful echoes of the past, frightful forecasts for the future, whispered, conspiratorial conversations, in voices too low and muffled for the meaning to be determined, mechanical sounds of unknown provenance, sounds unheard during the day and not associable with hospital operation. My emotions plummeting, I wanted to weep. I tried to. No use.

"Where's Marty?"

"He had to go to the hospital."

"Why?"

"He hurt his eye playing with the milk bottle. Don't you remember?"

"When will he come back?"

"Pretty soon. They will make his eye better and then he can come home."

"When?"

"Soon."

"Can I go and see him?"

"No."

"Why? Why can't I see him?"

"No children are allowed in the hospital. Go to bed."

"I just want to see him. I won't stay long. Please, mommy."

"I told you, it isn't allowed. Go to bed right now."

Upset, but obedient, I go to the bedroom. Turning the overhead light on, I undress. With one hand on the light switch, prepared to turn it off quickly and dive into the protective warmth of my bed, I look over at Marty's empty bed and feel myself beginning to cry. I don't want to cry. Mommy and Daddy will hear and be angry. The room looks huge, full of hidden threats. As the room clicks into darkness I fly into my bed, cocooning into the covers, huddling in the complete darkness, receiving some comfort from the spreading warmth. Gradually I uncover my head and peek in the direction of Marty's empty bed. Where is my Marty? Why isn't he here? Will he come back? When? The brittle, low voices of Mommy and Daddy drift into my room on the dim light emanating from the kitchen where they sit huddled, speaking in Russian and occasionally Yiddish. I know they are worried and that makes me think that Marty may never come back, but I can do nothing but hold tight to my child's prayer that he will come back. I cry softly until I fall asleep.

My room was a haven of stability and comfort. It was clean and bright and neat. The only sign of occupancy was my notebook and pen and the Kennedy novel I was reading lying on the table near the bed. My few belongings were hidden away in a small, ships cabin closet. Here, in this room, was order. After the wild flight of my post-operative, anesthesia-induced emotions, the sterile, uncomplicated atmosphere was what I needed. I walked around the room slowly. No demons anywhere to be seen. Luxuriantly, I removed my bathrobe and draped it on a nearby chair, turned off all but a reading light, wriggled into a comfortable position in bed and prepared to peacefully end the day reading.

I awoke the next morning hurting less, with the first real appetite in days. I showered, shaved and made some notes in a journal I had started to keep. I was hungry. Before and during breakfast, Kerry, a pleasant, middle-aged nurse, who came originally from the St. Louis area, repeated the offer of morphine. I declined again. With a noticeable degree of maternal exasperation she asked me if I was one of those men that had to show that I could take it. She faltered on the last words, deciding finally not to use a shortcut word such as macho or, perhaps, Rambo. I cut her last words short and assured her that I valued non pain over pain but that before I used any drug as strong as morphine I wanted to be certain that the anesthesia had disappeared from my system.

As I finished breakfast the room began filling with visitors. The orderly removing the breakfast tray, the young doctor taking my vital signs preparatory to approving my forthcoming discharge, a rabbi canvassing with an offer of spiritual comfort, the dietitian asking whether I'd be having lunch, a nurse asking whether I would need either a laxative or a prescription for morphine, all mingled with my visitors, bumping into and excusing each other, their voices rising in the competition to make themselves heard, quickly produced a din more resembling a subway car than a hospital room. Rappeport poked his head in and surveyed the scene wryly. Arline asked him, irreverently, if he considered that we had a *minyan* (the requisite ten men to conduct Jewish prayer services). Without hesitation he told her, "Not in my book."

The Brockelmans were introduced to Rappeport, and as soon as he discovered that Paul was a professor at the University of New Hampshire, Rappeport began interviewing him about the choice of schools for his son who, after a three year layoff, was interested in completing his master's in history. Instantly, Paul fell into the professorial mode, earnestly counseling Rappeport, who, in seconds became Paul's patient.

En masse we repeated the routine of the last two days and went to the Unit. Paul and Barbara, as well as others, were leaving shortly and would say goodbye to Marty and wish him well. Everyone put on his act: the same questions nervously asked and answered, variations of the same raucous jokes recently told, endless wishes for speedy recovery. People would have been more awkward had it not been for Marty. He was attentive to every comment and grateful for every good wish, alert and as sociable as possible. While the leave-taking was occurring, Vilunya was excitedly instructing me in how to read Marty's chart, the one I had been reading for days. I wondered whether it was a sign of stress or anxiety and I determined to pay attention to her in the forthcoming days. At last, the group flowed out of the Unit to go their separate ways, Arline and I to a farewell lunch with the Brockelmans after I checked out of the hospital.

Marty's danger was the greatest now. Two days after the transplant there was no evidence that the donated marrow was producing any effect. I was assured that there was nothing unusual about that. It could take another week or more before concrete signs of colonization appeared. While he waited, Marty was extremely sick with the effects of the conditioning regimen. He was holding very little food down and the vomiting was exhausting him. His hair was coming out in clumps.

I longed for quiet and a return to an orderly routine. Now that the visitors had gone, I intended to rest and nurse myself and become as calm as possible. Arline and I went immediately back to the hotel room where I rested, dozed and read. Arline, exhausted from the last two days, slept from mid-afternoon until the next morning.

I didn't sleep well and woke often during the night. I arose slowly next morning, dazed and hurting. I faxed a contract to Phoenix related to a sale of property. It had been weighing on my mind. The property was being sold at a huge loss, a salvage operation. It annoyed me but it was the best that could be done in the circumstances: a building we had bought during the halcyon days, leased at the time for far more than it would bring now. Realistically, I knew the deal I had just accepted was the best I could do, but it irked me.

My pelvic area and tailbone ached fiercely. I was sorry I had not accepted the morphine. Out of sorts, I changed the dressing that covered the punctures, and, unsteadily, went to the breakfast area of the hotel to consume their cardboard continental breakfast..

Marty was sitting up and writing when I arrived at the Unit. He was still coughing up clots of mucous. Although he looked listless, he said he had been reading and exercising a short time before. His exercise was walking in place and swinging his arms. He could venture to the end of his tether, the lines attached to the catheters in his chest.

We spoke for a few minutes. I saw the distance between us reflected in Marty's eyes. The plastic curtain formed an ever-growing barrier between his daily experience and that of every visitor, including Vilunya and me. Vilunya told me much later she thought she saw contempt in his eyes, sometimes directed at her. I hadn't noticed Marty looking at her differently from the rest of us, and, in any event, contempt didn't seem the right characterization. It appeared to me the look of staring across a widening gulf. His suffering, and his hearing loss related to the heavy radiation and chemotherapy, made it difficult for him to hear the muffled voices on the other side of the curtain or read the ambiguous expressions of those who wished him well but couldn't bear the sight of him in his present circumstances. That removal, that withdrawal, shows in his eyes,

There, in the stillness of his solitary condition, he thinks of his past and wonders whether he will have a future, and if he does, what it will be like. Marty is and has been, husband, father, student, merchant sailor, soldier, field anthropologist, professor, author, advocate for the voiceless, political advisor, brother, son. Now, sealed in his room, he aspires only to be survivor. He has neither wife nor mother, child nor brother. He is alone. His wasted, weakened body will give him no protection or strength. He must build strength from his will. No one can help him except the medical technology he has already had the use of. He is at the hinge moment of his survival. Alone, patient and unafraid, he must do and think what sustains him, without regard for any convention or custom, without regard for anyone's feelings.

I thought of discussing these things with him, but I didn't feel strong enough. I resolved to think of things to do to draw Marty to us, to prevent him from falling so deeply into isolation that returning will be difficult. We spoke vacantly until his treatment began and then I withdrew with a cup of coffee and Marty's chart to wait to resume the visit.

The pregnant young woman was visiting her husband, Ray, in the next room. Perched on the high stool and facing him through the curtain, her head and shoulders, as well as her husband's, were in my line of sight. Their conversation was muted at first, the usual faint buzz affected by patients and visitors, designed neither to intrude upon nor or be heard by people in adjoining rooms, and out of respect, usually censored out of comprehension by those within earshot.

Ray's voice grew louder, clearer to me even in the other room, more insistent, angrier. I could see his head bobbing as he replied to her. He was admonishing her to cease dwelling on the death of her father. She countered by telling him, in a needy voice, what he already knew: that her relationship with her father was an unhappy one, that they had not spoken to each other in the two years prior to his death. He scolded her, ordered her, with disgust in his voice, to put it behind her. Uncomfortably, neither one spoke for perhaps a minute.

"The dog has loose stools again."

"Make sure he has plenty of water and only dry food", he said in a slightly softened tone.

They lapsed into a silence that exaggerated the sound of the everblaring TV.

"Do you want to sleep now?" It was a familiar phrase. Although put in the interrogatory it was a declaration that the visitor wanted to flee. Ray made no immediate reply.

"Have you started getting the house ready for me? It's got to be clean, as close to sterile as possible."

"I've begun wiping everything down. The upstairs bedroom will be ready for you. Have they said when you can come home?"

"As soon as a couple of weeks if nothing goes wrong."

They sat in tense silence. A quiz show was heard. She must have again raised the subject of the difficulty of her father's death in a voice too low for me to hear.

"Stop it! Put it behind you. You can't keep thinking about it. Why can't you deal with it?" He was almost shouting, his lean and muscular upper body elevated as if poised to strike at her, cobra-like, through the plastic curtain.

"Because you know why, because we didn't speak the last two years," she said resignedly, defenseless. "I have good days and bad days – like everyone."

Disturbed by what I had heard eavesdropping, I left the Unit quickly and went to the cafeteria. The sight and smell of that food, with which I was too familiar, robbed me of appetite. I walked through the teeming lobby, jostling with the streaming crowd and left the building and into the blazing sun and wilting humidity. Across the street from the hospital several kinds of Chinese food, Mexican, Korean, Southern barbecue, Vietnamese, delicatessen were sold from wagons beckoning the hungry with their sights and smells.

This was where the menial staff of the hospital dined out. Except for the occasional doctor, intern or resident, distinguished by dress and conspicuous stethoscope, the rest of the sidewalk patrons pushed gurneys and did the housekeeping of the hospital. The air was full of raucous, appreciative sounds, riots of laughter, deep-throated sexual offers and coquettishly indignant refusals, overly dramatized anger at workplace injustices, loose limbed movement that unkinked the body, and pleasurable consumption of the wagon food, noisily washed down with soda pop in bottles and cans.

Surrounding this scene were high rise buildings of institutional anonymity inside of which the business and the science of medicine was conducted. Research labs, teaching facilities, administration, and in the hospital itself, care of human beings, of patients. Inside, the atmosphere was gray and subdued. Inside, was leukemia. Outside, during the lunch hour, the ground shook with life and freedom. I was glad that Marty's window did not afford a view of the throbbing scene I was in the midst of. It would have been too cruel for him to crane his neck at the end of his tether and see what he could not be part of.

Marty was alert and glad to see me. We talked for a while mostly about how he felt. He had slept well after a dose of Demerol. I scrubbed and suited up to enter his room. We exercised together – walking out the length of his tether and back and marching in place. He settled in his bed gratefully after the short exercise session and fell asleep quickly.

It was the fourth day after the transplant, too early to see any results. Nobody spoke of the lurking fear: infection. So far, he seemed relatively healthy, no fevers, rashes or respiratory complications. The worst of the nausea and vomiting seemed to be over. Even-spirited, content to wait passively, he didn't express impatience either with his circumstances or with those around him.

I delivered Arline to a health club and stopped on the way to the hospital to buy two more Kennedy books. I loved Ironweed and was eager to read more.

Marty's latest blood test showed a nucleated red blood cell. Since only immature, recently formed red cells have nuclei, there was strong suspicion that it had been produced by the donated marrow. Still no sign yet of what we were all looking for – white blood cells.

Arline and I had made arrangements to spend two days visiting my cousin, Ed Victor, who had invited us to his summer home in Long Island. Vilunya would be with Marty while I was gone and the next week she would go home for a couple of days while I stayed. I was nervous about leaving but thrilled at the prospect of getting away from the hospital for a while.

Vilunya, Arline and I had dinner that night. I dined on marrow building food, steak and wine. We were all more relaxed than we had been in some time, but I could clearly see how stressed Vilunya was. Although not given to displaying emotion, she wept briefly when we spoke of Marty. The evening passed pleasantly. We spoke mostly of our children. The wine loosened us all and we gave the outward appearance of having a normal evening, but try as we did to enjoy the dinner for itself, Marty sat at the table with us. Vilunya asked Arline many questions about Asa, the first of his generation. Her cheeks glowed and her eyes shone with warmth at the news of her great-nephew.

There was a great hubbub in the Unit the next morning. Kathryn, a baby at the time, had been transplanted with marrow donated by a young English woman, a total stranger. Now, not yet three years old, she and her parents were brought face to face with the donor. Kathryn was scampering wildly around the Unit, opening and closing doors and drawers, loudly greeting everyone she encountered. Kathryn's parents were nervously eyeing those around them as if looking for some clue as how to act. The young English woman was standing near the parents, sporadically conversing with them, observing everything carefully, somewhat bewildered by the commotion. She was in her late twenties, slender and attractive, plainly dressed, the mother of three, who had registered as a donor and was a close match to Kathryn. Rappeport was ostensibly presiding over the structureless scene. He withdrew a slight distance and, with tears glistening in his eyes, watched the nurses hug and kiss their former little patient.

There was a policy at the Bone Marrow Transplant Unit that recipients and anonymous donors were not permitted to become acquainted with each other until one year after the procedure. The reason was obvious. It would be an unfair burden on the donor to learn of the death of the recipient. Rappeport conducted a press conference in front of the hospital to tell Kathryn's story. His remarks were given newspaper coverage. It was good advertising for the hospital and the BMT Unit.

I asked him later how Kathryn was kept inside a room without doors. He told me that even at her young age, and with as much pain as she was experiencing, she never tried to leave her room, as if she knew that staying in the room was her only chance for life. While Kathryn and her family were in the Unit we all watched her with interest. She was proof that a cure was possible. Not a cheerful statistic or an anecdote, but a sweet little girl, active and normal in every outward aspect, restored to health. Marty craned his neck to see the festivities. We were all buoyed by the sight of Kathryn.

Marty appeared to have white blood cells. That morning's blood count showed 200 per cubic centimeter. A normal count is 10,000. An infection can produce counts of 15,000 to 20,000. In contrast 200 is the equivalent of zero, I told myself. It's not enough to help him fight disease. It might not even be a real count. But with a thrill I had to struggle to suppress, I knew that it could be the first sign that Marty was engrafting. I quietly asked Dr. Ahmad what it meant. He said it was too early to tell, that conclusions should not be drawn from this one reading, that if the counts increased over the next number of days we could conclude that Marty was indeed engrafting. I read his comments as designed to not raise my hopes unrealistically. It seemed like standard doctor to family of patient fare. I accepted it willingly. The next few days would tell. In the meantime we won't tip the gods off. By the time they learn of the success of the transplant they won't be able to undo it. We'll sneak it right past them.

Vilunya came bounding down the hall, exultantly declaring the transplant a success.

"Did you see the counts? He has 200 white cells."

"Yes, I saw them. Nobody knows what it means yet."

"It means he's engrafting. Yesterday no white cells. Today 200. They had to come from the transplant, from you."

I wanted to punch her out. I wanted to gag her. Didn't she know she was endangering everything? She couldn't stop smiling and silently clapping her hands. She insisted on dragging me over to the chart and showing me the .02 along the line that read WBC for today. She pointed out that for days, since the full effect of the radiation, his white blood count didn't register at all. I felt myself going sour. It was not that I didn't want to believe that Marty was engrafting. I desperately did not want my hopes raised only to have Marty slip away from me. Imagining that felt like death to me. I broke away from Vilunya as soon as I could and wandered around the hospital for a while, confused and angry.

The turnoff to the village of San Sebastian de Teitipac was unmarked. It lay along the paved road between Oaxaca and Tlacolula. It was not on the way to any place. The road ended at the Teitipac villages. You had to know the way and have a reason for going there. Marty, who had been conducting an ethnographic study for a year, had both.

Arline and I had arrived in Oaxaca that day for a month-long visit. When Marty met us at the airport he told us he had to pick up Vilunya, who was in the village. Arline stayed at their house in the city and I accompanied Marty.

His Land Rover sighed resignedly as Marty shifted down to turn onto the dirt road that led to the village. The next ten miles would take thirty or forty minutes. The road showed no sign of having been bladed. Formidable rocks were revealed as the powdered dirt blew away. Not many cars or trucks used it. The vehicular traffic was mostly the soft drink truck and the occasional pickup truck. Horses and burros conveyed more people than cars.

Marty was excitedly telling me what to expect at the village, which was in the third day of the fiesta of the Patron Saint, the most important celebration of the year. The early evening dying winter light created long shadows in the road, some of them indistinguishable from the sharp, upthrusted rocks. Marty parked at the edge of the dusty plaza, where, an electrical cord strung with naked light bulbs illuminated the musicians and the remaining dancing celebrants. On the periphery were small stands, open to the weather, with food for the guests.

Vilunya was one of four or five singles and a like number of couples, swaying to the labored sounds of the five-piece brass band. She was shuffling rhythmically; her eyes closed, her arms at her sides, the pale yellow electrical light accentuating the perspiration glow of her face. It was obvious that the present day's fiesta activities were coming to a close, the musicians dutifully completing their service, the celebrants dancing their last. We stood for a while just watching Vilunya dancing in the midst of the villagers. Taller and fairer than any of her fellow dancers, she seemed completely at her ease. In a minute or two she noticed us, and with a cry of "Saul," she ran over to embrace me. Villagers gave us curious looks as we exchanged greetings. She was exhilarated.

"Isn't this great? I'm so glad you're here. I'm falling off my feet. I'm ready to go home," she said, breathlessly.

It was apparent that she was equally ready to stay, that she loved being there. An elderly, stooped woman walked past us slowly. Vilunya took her gently by the arm, drew her into our group and, bending slightly, loudly introduced me. I extended my hand, preparing a greeting in my rudimentary Spanish. The old lady grasped my fingers with her bird's claw and quickly drew my hand toward her, kissing the back of it. Somewhat stunned by my first Zapotec greeting, I reciprocated awkwardly.

Marty and Vilunya took me around the plaza explaining everything and introducing me to the villagers. We went from stand to stand greeting people who offered us food. Vilunya animatedly explained what was in each pot. I asked her why she was carrying a small backpack. We were standing in front of a large pot containing a pig's head floating in a sea of yellowish fat. Vilunya explained, "It's rude to refuse food, but it's perfectly good manners to take it home with you rather than eat it on the spot."

A short, dark man with deep wrinkles around his eyes approached us. Marty turned to face him.

"Don Adelaido, I would like to present my brother, Saul, from the United States." His small, but powerful, hand swiftly brought my hand to his mouth. He straightened and looked at us, alternately, with amazement.

"You look alike."

"We're brothers," said Marty

"But you look exactly alike."

"Well, we're twins," explained Marty, using a slightly ambiguous word to describe us.

"But you look like one person," Don Adelaido repeated, dumbfounded, looking at one and then the other.

"We are twins."

Don Adelaido's mouth fell open. His eyes widened with astonishment. "But you both survived."

The trip to Long Island, on three ferryboats, to visit my cousin Ed, was a balm. Feeling the ocean breeze, cool and free, began to loosen the tight grip of the fetid interior of the hospital. Marty was on my mind constantly, but without the immediacy of the atmosphere of the Unit, with its charts and serious nurses and gravely countenanced doctors and sorrow-laden visitors. No voice boomed periodically over the hospital intercom announcing impending tragedy, no ghastly, gray patients, the life ebbing out of them, being wheeled past me. Just the grind of the ferry machinery, the *shush* of the mild waves parted by the boat and the scream of gulls scanning everywhere for food and disapproving our intrusion on their domain. I was happy to see Arline standing at the rail, her eyes half shut, smiling with joy at the wind blowing over her. It gave me a feeling of optimism. Although, superstitiously, I hadn't said it aloud to Vilunya, I was confident Marty was engrafting. Only slightly beneath that optimism was the guilty realization that perhaps the best part of the next two days of desporting myself in Hamptonia, was that I wouldn't have to see Marty, to watch him suffer.

Ed and his sons, Adam and Ivan, met us at the last ferry landing. Amid the kisses and hugs I could see in their faces that I looked frail and pained to them. Within minutes Ed was arraying plans for the two days, indicating clearly that would do his best to distract me with enjoyments. The time passed swiftly and pleasurably.

I overdid it those two days, knowingly. My body, just being used to drag me around the hospital corridors, felt useless, and I wanted some proof of my vitality. I swam and played tennis and we went speeding through the sound in Ed's boat. My bandages, soaked in water and drenched in sweat, melted into my skin. My hips ached ferociously and the pain shot down my leg. I exulted in the pain. Let the damn things ache. At least they'll carry me around the tennis court and propel me around in the water. Beneath the pain I was satisfied I could feel some muscle tone, a harbinger of healing. I thought, with a sick feeling, of Marty's doctor telling him not to worry about his weight loss, that he was only losing muscle mass.

We returned to New Haven late at night and I arrived at the hospital mid-morning of the next day. Although the two day respite was a great tonic for me, I was oddly pleased to be back in what were now familiar surroundings.

Marty was engrafting! I was secretly sure of it, and his count seemed to be confirming it. Vilunya had been right, I admitted sheepishly to myself. He had 300 white cells today. More importantly, it was the third, maybe fourth day in a row of discernible counts. When I asked the people on the Unit, nurses and doctors, what the counts meant, I still received carefully hedged answers as before, but this time I detected a suppressed excitement. Content with those answers, and struggling to control my rising optimism, I went in to see Marty.

Despite his lifting himself energetically up on his pillows as I approached his room, Marty's "hi" was a falling tone. His expression was pained.

"Not doing too well?"

"No, not really."

"Anything go wrong? Are you feeling badly? Any change in the counts?"

Marty looked away for a time before he answered. "Everything seems to be the same as it was when you left. The counts, if anything, are a little improved. I'm obsessing again. I'm probably a little depressed. I'm glad to see you. How did it go?"

"Did you feel that I abandoned you?"

"Yeah, I probably do, or did. I know that you needed a little time away just as Vilunya and Leah do, but just laying here, all alone, my mind starts racing and imagining all kinds of dark things. I guess I was a little jealous, too."

I knew he didn't want to feel as he did. He expressed himself in an elemental way, just telling me his feelings, without varnish, without guile. It seemed to do him some good to say it. It didn't make me feel guilty to hear it. I put one hand through the plastic gauntlet. He grasped it and we held that position for a while, a motionless handshake. "It was good for me to get away. Ed couldn't have been nicer. He had planned a round of diverting activities. I enjoyed the time, although my mind wasn't all there. It feels good to be back here with you. Aside from all that, how're you doing?" We smiled broadly at each other, putting an end to that discussion..

We didn't discuss the engrafting progress. The time or two I mentioned the increasing counts, in a tone intended to be dry and factual, or Vilunya, in an enthusiastic, victorious tone, Marty barely acknowledged that we were speaking to him. Part of his reaction was caused by his painfully low physical condition which invariably produced depressed behavior. Part of it was that Marty shared my primitive attitude about declaring victory before it was certain. Too much was at stake. His limited capacity for disappointments made it wiser not to create wild expectations that, when not realized, would be crushing defeats.

Vilunya, on the other hand, needed to have her spirits uplifted. That Marty's white count had risen from 200 to 300 as of this day, August 21, 1993, was a fact. 300 was better than 200, 200 better than zero. Tomorrow might reveal another fact, a continuation of progress or a setback. That was for tomorrow. Today the news could rightfully be called good and Vilunya was going to revel in it because it nourished her, gave her courage. Of everyone involved in Marty's illness, his family, children, friends and colleagues, only Vilunya had been there from the beginning and had been witness to every frightening and tragic moment. She received the bad news at the same time as he did, beginning with the first diagnosis over twenty years ago as well as the step-by-step announcements of his deteriorating health. She waited for the doctors to tell her whether he survived his emergency surgery, she rode with him in the ambulance, she sat with him in the emergency rooms. As Marty's spirits plunged, it was Vilunya who listened to his despair as she saw him wasting away, as she saw the pain she could not alleviate. How many times in those many, many, moments, throughout those years, did she wonder whether Marty would die and leave her alone? How could she survive, this frail orphan from Poland, without the person she loved and could always count on? And even more vexing; how long could she care for Marty while watching his suffering? It was apparent by now that, even assuming the success of the transplant, his convalescence would be long, and probably difficult. The description, in my thoughts, of Vilunya as a "frail orphan from Poland" was overblown. I thought of her that way only when she was at her lowest, hurting and unsure of the future. She was certainly not frail. Having survived her childhood hinted at the deep reserves she had. She would find the strength to do more than survive.

In some respect it is easier to be the sufferer than the onlooker/caretaker. The sufferer has the first hand knowledge of when changes occur, how severe symptoms are. In the case of a catastrophic ailment such as Marty's, the disease dominates the plans of the household, its schedule. The threat of an outbreak of a symptom overhangs every plan made. Communication becomes desperately difficult. How can Marty precisely articulate the severity of what he may be feeling, find the proper scale to describe the pain, or other symptom, in a way that conveys clinically to Vilunya, the current situation? Does he exaggerate, either to allay her fears or to gain more sympathy than his present state warrants? How can he explain to her that irrespective of the conventional medical explanation, a certain pain or enervation, or other symptom even subtler, may to him, in a depressed condition, foretell his death? Does she learn to read him, to interpret what he tells her in such a way that she becomes able to weigh his statements and arrive at accurate conclusions? Or does her imagination intrude in those formulations, the demons hissing malevolently in her ear, increasing her fear and foreboding in those exchanges?

Vilunya did what she had to do for herself. Essentially a cheerful person, she latched onto any scrap of good news, especially now, at this most dangerous moment for Marty. Like a person shackled at the ankle to a heavy ball, she drew enough strength from good news to hurl the ball forward so that when it reached the end of its tether, it dragged her forward. That couldn't always work. From time to time, especially during periods when Marty looked like he was sinking, Vilunya's cheer and resolve and certainty broke down. She would retreat like a bewildered animal and silently try to restore herself.

August 22nd was our 59th birthday. Vilunya planned a party in the Unit. She scouted out a bakery in the vicinity that met her standards and commissioned an elaborate cake. Her cheeks had high color as she bustled happily around the Unit presenting us with cake and soft drinks and herding us near Marty to sing happy birthday to him. Marty accepted the gaiety with a dull smile. He had slept well the night before as a result of a new sleeping pill. I thought that he was probably still in a drugged haze. The nurses were jolly, genuinely happy for the change in atmosphere. Marty received congratulatory phone calls. Rita and Randy appeared and reservedly joined the celebration. Randy scanned the room, observing the therapeutic installations and looking Marty over with a diagnostic eye. Rappeport offered his congratulations on both the birthday and the cake. The brief celebration died away as Marty fell asleep. His chart showed that his white count had doubled, to six hundred.

The next morning Marty's white count was one thousand. I asked Wendy, the head nurse and Dr. Ahmad what they thought. Both said that my marrow was active. Finding the answer ambiguous, I asked Wendy pointedly if it meant that Marty was engrafting. Looking me firmly in the eye she told me it did mean that he was engrafting. Rappeport came by and I asked him the same question. He verified what Wendy and Haroon had said and told me he was especially pleased with the monocyte production. He said, with a sly grin, but with genuine enthusiasm, that our mother would be proud.

It was sinking in to my mind. The process that had begun ten days before was working well. Little bits of information, of evidence, had been accumulating, building the case that the transplant was probably successful. I dared then to ask Rappeport when he thought Marty could go home. It was the test for me. If these early results were inconclusive, or worse, negative, he would caution me to not get too excited and declare that it was premature to talk of going home. Instead, he told me matter-of-factly that, barring any other complications, Marty could go home when his neutrophils were at 1,000. Neutrophils are the percentage of segs and *bands* (whatever they are) in the white blood count. That total would be

217

used as a percentage of his white cells. If, for instance, Marty's white cell count went to 4,000 and his *segs* and *bands* totaled 30%, his neutrophil count would be 1,200, more than enough. It was still too early for me to celebrate, but, now, finally, I believed it was happening.

I realized, with an anxious pang, that I would be leaving in a week. Arline would leave in a day or two for a day's visit in New York and then on to Cincinnati to spend a few more days before returning to Phoenix. Marty was lethargic most of the time. He was still intermittently sick at his stomach and almost constantly profoundly fatigued. He still seemed only mildly interested in his increasing counts, acknowledging them with little discussion. I determined that I was going to behave as if I were certain that the success of the transplant was now a settled matter, the counts merely the indicator of the speed of his recovery. I brought him fresh VCR movies every couple of days. I tried to talk of the wider world, of current events, politics, literature. Marty was tolerant of such talk, but not engaged. Those conversations withered away quickly and deadened the air.

I spent one afternoon alone, driving around New Haven, looking at buildings designed by world famous architects. New Haven undoubtedly has more buildings per capita built by easily recognizable architects than any city in the world. It was a feast, from the formality of the Kahn museums to the playful Venturi fire station to the dynamic Saarinen skating rink. They went on forever. I stopped after I had seen perhaps 15 or 20 of them, and returned refreshed, to stroll through the Yale campus on the way back to Marty.

Marty was engrafting. Everyone, in his own way, said it. His white count was increasing daily. By the 28th of August it was 4,700, his neutrophils approaching 40%, enough to permit him to go home. But the higher his count went the lower his spirits seemed to sink. His hair was still coming out in handfuls, the wisps of hair and patches of scalp unevenly framing his face, giving him a wild and scabrous appearance. His hair loss meant that the chemotherapy and radiation were still killing cells in his body at the same time the new marrow was creating new blood cells. What a strange and horrible sensation it must have been to feel part of the body dying while in the same body new life is forming. It happens all the time, of course, in a healthy body, old cells die and are eliminated while new cells are formed. But I imagine that to be a slow and subtle process, one that can't be felt. What Marty was experiencing was the acceleration and magnification of that process, a rampant intensification of it, something that didn't exist in nature and until the last eyeblink in the history of human kind, never experienced.

He also had a fever, initially accompanied by a light rash. Rappeport thought it could be a touch of Graft Versus Host Disease but because of the perfect match between Marty and me, more properly called Graft Versus Leukemia. If it really were the latter it would be a good thing. It was never fully determined whether he had graft versus anything. The fever was troublesome. They made cultures to identify the infectious agent and gave up after several unsuccessful attempts. The fever gradually reduced and, it seemed to me, his spirits rose in direct proportion to that improvement.

It was apparent to me by now that I would leave New Haven before Marty was to be released from the hospital. It was time for me to go. I awoke in pain almost every morning, my hips and lower back aching, and dragged myself to the hospital. Some mornings I longed to be away from the entire experience: not to have to see Marty's pain, not to have to feel my own, not to have to smell the decay of the hospital corridors, masked clumsily by the chemical deodorants. On the way to the hospital, even after the previous day's impressive improvement, my mind teemed with potential setbacks and tragedies. Usually before I saw Marty I would look at his chart and see the gains he had made in the last 24 hours. And yet, when I would see Marty through the plastic curtain more often than not his expression was sad and defeated. I knew that he was not daring to trust the good news completely and he didn't have the strength to put on a cheerful mask. He was still throwing up from time to time and his fevers had not completely gone; a fact that troubled everyone, especially Marty. Rappeport told Marty that, if not for the fever, he could go home in a week or ten days.

Marty was beginning to believe it. He became interested in the preparations to the house that would have to be made before he could return to Lexington. The house had to be as free as possible from molds and fungi that could possibly infect him. It was determined after considerable discussion that Vilunya and Leah would store away many furnishings and decorations in an effort to make the house easier to keep clean. In a 200-year-old house that was no small consideration. Then they would hire a service to scour the house clean from basement to attic. Marty's interest in these arrangements flagged after the first few exchanges, in which he gleaned the essentials. The detailed discussion did not interest him. He seemed to be considering having his passport stamped, to rejoin the land he had left. He wasn't sure if it was for a visit or to resume residence. The doctors had said that the time for recovery from the BMT, that is, to be able to resume the life he had before the transplant, could be from six to eighteen months.

Whereas I was ready to declare victory and retire from the field of combat feeling righteous and self-satisfied, Marty pondered what his life would be like over the next months and longer: whether he would ever fully regain his vitality, how diminished his life might become, would he ever be able to travel to Central America again, to the unhealthy places of his life long interest.

I awoke the next morning, a Sunday, feeling better. It was still early and I decided to treat myself to a proper breakfast. Though an overnight rain had washed the streets clean, the overall aspect of the business district in which I walked looked ruined and dazed rather than clean. Only two kinds of people were to be seen that morning. The kind belonging to the city, those who had no escape: pensioners who retire too early and rise too early and those wearied by drugs or alcohol and lack of sleep, contemplating the early morning through sick, defeated, eyes. The others were students associated with Yale, getting an early start on the school year. Those scrubbed youngsters moved with nervous purpose, slightly defensive in the unaccustomed environment. Some were jogging or speed walking. A few girls, walking alone, strode purposefully, their thin purse straps bisecting their tee-shirted chests.

I ate at a small Greek restaurant, familiar-looking from the Brooklyn of my youth. After a five minute wait in the dirty vestibule, I was seated at a counter and gave my order to a bored, inattentive elderly waitress, who barely turning her head to spare me the full volume of her voice, bellowed out my order in what seemed like a mixture of English and Greek to the sweating cook five feet away. It was exactly what I wanted; eggs fried in grease, overly crisp bacon, toasted white bread and strong coffee. It felt like a breakfast on the road, a respite from energetic activity and it left me feeling enlivened, in the full thrum of activity of the real world, the world I would soon rejoin.

Marty was blue, exhausted, slightly woozy. Although his counts continued to improve, he had no energy. His cheeks were aflame, despite the fact that his fever was low grade and trending lower. They still don't know if he has an infection – they haven't been able to culture anything. They speculated as to whether he had an allergic reaction, perhaps to the antibiotics or a touch of GVHD. He is still throwing up periodically. He was not getting much nutrition.

Vilunya comes by a little later. I can sense the strain in her speech and in her demeanor. She will be leaving for Boston in the morning. She desperately needs the few days respite. The thought of the short liberty buoys her at the moment, but to acknowledge it frankly might appear to be disloyal to Marty. Part of her wants to stay, the other parts need to go. Guilt is subsumed in the lifesaving need to draw fresh air into her lungs, not the air of sickness and suffering. I think I know what she is feeling. I feel it myself.

At the end of the day Vilunya and I join Rita and Randy to have pizza. After the meal Vilunya and I say goodbye to each other. I will have left New Haven by the time she returns. It is the most concrete of the events leading up to my departure. First Arline left and now Vilunya. In a couple of days I will leave. As we kiss and hug goodbye, Vilunya thanks me for coming. I mutter something. By unspoken agreement there will be no emotion demonstrated now. This parting is not significant, just another event in a long continuum, leading certainly to Marty's full restoration. His release from the hospital should just be regarded as an episode.

I went back to the hospital. Marty and I watched a movie together. We didn't talk much. Although I felt a little better about leaving him now than I did a week ago, I was still worried about his future. What do all those undiagnosed symptoms mean? Are they serious? Can they be resolved easily, or they a potential constellation of unforeseen problems related to the still experimental BMT procedure, the outcome of which are still in doubt?

The next morning, as if on cue, Marty was looking and feeling better. He had slept well and held down his breakfast. His eyes looked clear and alert. I rejoiced. Marty was not going to let me leave him carrying the image of him drawn and suffering. Rappeport, also as if on cue, confirmed that he was not concerned with the slight fever or the light rash. Providing nothing changed for the worse, Marty could be released in another week.

I scrubbed and went into his room so that we might be able to visit without raising our voices to be heard through the plastic. Marty was sitting in his bed, erect and alert. We gave each other a bulky embrace.

"This will be your last visit in my room."

"Yeah. I won't miss it. I'm sure you won't."

I won't miss it, but…" He paused, molding the thought into words.

"It's kept me alive until now. Apparently until I engrafted. The transplant is successful, isn't it?"

"Yes, it is successful." I met his eyes directly. Because my mouth and nose were covered by the surgical mask he had to see in my eyes that I believed it to be the truth. "The Rapman says so, Haroon says so, and all the nurses say so. Your chart confirms it. There is no doubt about it so far as I am concerned."

Marty accompanied my presentation with a slight rhythmic nodding of his head, his eyes fastened on mine, reading me. He turned away, pretending to make some adjustment in the lines leading to the I.V. tree standing outside the plastic wall. There was something else.

"I've written you a letter. I'm not quite sure it's coherent."

The thought of receiving a letter from Marty represented a proof to me that I was indeed leaving the next day. It opened the gate containing my emotions, and like a canal lock, I could feel a liquid welling inside. We looked at each other for a long time, in silence.

"How do you feel about my leaving?" The question was as proforma as it was obligatory, a ritual. I had asked Marty that question before and, though I couldn't know it then, I would ask it again in the future. It was, at the same time, asking Marty for the frankest evaluation of his condition and for his permission for me to leave.

His face forced a smile, a protection against tears. "You know, I want you to stay, but I know, you have to go..." His voice cracked and his tears came, reluctantly releasing me, acknowledging that he felt out of danger. We both wept softly, averting our eyes from the other to permit a recovery sufficient to be able to continue. There was something else.

"This has been so hard, and the future is still so uncertain that I'm not sure I have the will to fight any more, to get well." He said it without much emotion. The doctors didn't tell him how hard it would be – they simply didn't know. Marty knew. He knew from listening to his weakened body.

"Until now, Marty, you've shown an abundance of will. You battled for survival for at least the last two years. Without that ferocious will of yours you wouldn't be what you are today, a survivor of leukemia. The worst is behind you, *mano*. What you need now is rest and recuperation. No goals, no schedules – just rest."

It sounded like the truth to me, but I couldn't be certain that it was. Neither could Marty. If I, in Marty's situation, had expressed my fear of lacking the will to survive Marty would have made the same speech to me and it would have comforted me.

Marty handed me the letter he had written to me. It was on two sheets of rumpled and slightly stained paper. I was not expecting it yet. It was difficult to read because of the tremulous hand. I began reading it, skipping over parts that were not readily decipherable. We cried as I read.

Sat. 28 Agosto
early morning
Dear Sauly,

As your stay ends here, I am aware of how important it has been to me. And I'm pleased that your knowledge of the evolution of the case leaves you less stressed and anxious about its outcome.

I awoke this morning so deeply imbedded in a dream that it still surrounds me. It concerned an alternate form of health care where a team of young, sprightful, well trained people would make suggestions and carry them out, arguing they could not have cost more and may be useful. So today I'm going to ask for a cold bath to chill those inflamed, red, itchy parts. Sleeping will be the next hurdle. The fact that it was a dream matters little, it's the ideas and initiatives that emerge.

This experience has been so marginalizing and isolating (a la Murphy) and I've contributed by withdrawing. But I hope I've turned a corner now. Instead of nodding yes or no to utterances muffled by masks or curtain and showing the nurses and docs that I don't have to strain to hear them because I don't care what they're saying, I'm now ready to launch suggestions that come from my felt need to start being positive about the curing and healing process.

While all the years of being a CLLer have given me a certain edge about how to live, nothing has prepared me for this hospital stay. It's more like an expulsion from society and, hopefully, a full return in a different status. A rite de passage. But, unlike the primitives who are clear about the status left behind and the new one being entered, here it is I and a few intimates who can be privy to this. I had been treating the transplant as an interruption, but it is much more. It must be a redefinition. Since I feel so way out and distant from every thing at least I can return somewhat different if I want.

I will certainly come back to you. Our twinship, cubhood, are like attractants, forces of nature. Perhaps more though is our adult friendship, our ability to persevere through momentary rough spots. How wonderful to be friends with your cub.

My job is to give thought to the return. I have no notion at this moment what that means. Surviving each day is enough. My handwriting gives an idea of that.

But back I'll come, dear manito, maybe with a different paint job, maybe not. We have more twinning to do and I'm anxious to begin.

Marty

I told him that I was not leaving with a heavy heart. I told him that he and I would survive, that I loved him. He told me he loved me. We embraced and I left his room to remove the sterile garb for the last time.

I awoke early with a start, my head and stomach aching. I was to leave today to catch an afternoon flight from New York to Cincinnati. Before I fell asleep the night before I carefully scheduled the day's activities, assigning times to every task that lay before me. I wanted the day to be full to counter the sadness of leaving, full enough to truncate saying goodbye to Marty but not so full as to either neglect some important arrangement or to be forced to rush my leave-taking. I flew out of bed and standing tensely in the middle of the room my mind flooded with the most intensely trivial of details as I engaged in what I told myself was planning.

Should I shower first and then pack? If I did that would the packing, combined with my nervousness produce a foul sweat that would require me to shower again? If I packed first could I take steps that would guarantee to remind me not to forget my toilet kit, which would then have to be the last thing packed? Should I have breakfast first? Aside from the clothes I had set aside to travel in did I have clothes presentable enough to go to the breakfast room of the hotel? Was I hungry enough to eat breakfast? Should I eat breakfast even if I wasn't hungry to avoid being famished later in the day or should I just have a glass of juice from the fridge in the room and maybe brew a cup of tea?

I opened the refrigerator door and as I reached for the juice my eye rested on the almost empty bottle of gin next to it. The thought of a deep draught of straight gin and the calming it would afford appealed strongly to me, and as my hand moved ambiguously in its direction I pictured myself as the morally honest but unsuccessful cheap detective dosing himself with the hair of the dog to begin the day and I laughed out loud. That settled it for me. I poured a glass of orange juice, put some water to boil for tea and jumped into the shower.

Marty looked good, genuinely good, better I told myself, than he could have willed himself to look to make my leaving easier. His face was not red. His eyes were brighter and he seemed to have more energy. He told me he ate his entire breakfast and held it down. Describing his plan to resume the light exercise program he had started a week or so ago, he felt at a turning point. He would go home soon and he was taking positive steps to accomplish that. My dear Marty was also feigning some strength and enthusiasm and, in general, health. That was as it should be. Some feigning was good for both of us.

We spoke about Leah, with whom I had had dinner the night before, about her life, about her last, hard year. We talked of other matters, family, friends, even touched on politics, with no sad reference to my leaving in an hour. Mom had called before I arrived during Marty's ablutions. I returned the call, spoke to her for a minute or two and Marty continued the conversation while I went to say goodbye to Carol and Ray and the nurses. I heard Marty telling Mom how good he felt and how soon he thought he would go home.

Carol was almost in tears. Although we had spoken little these past weeks, we had been aware of each other. Her illness was sapping her strength. The red rash from the GVHD covered her body and her pain was carved into her face. The handshake through the plastic turned into an embrace of hands. She told me she will leave as soon as the GVHD clears up and emotionally wished Marty and the rest of our family well.

Ray, with whom, I also had only exchanged perfunctory greetings and abbreviated conversation, wanted to talk. He told me how hard it was for him. Even from the vantage point of the soon anticipated end of his suffering, he confided with some emotion, that he probably would not have elected to do it if he had known how awful it turned out to be. He allowed that twice he almost walked out of the room during his stay, a move that would have meant his death. Somewhat surprised by the frankness of what he has revealed to me, a stranger, he signaled the end of our talk. We exchanged good wishes and a brief plastic handshake.

Rappeport is nowhere to be found. I determine to write to him. Haroon bids me a good trip and suggests that I should be confident about Marty. His manner is British, helpful, just the correct side of familiar. The nurses on duty today know I am leaving and are grouped near their station. I bid them all goodbye and express my thanks. They have performed this ritual many times and try to make the moment business-like, but the compassion they bring to their job, that contributes to making them the great caregivers they are, shines forth from their faces. Each nurse's hand characterizes her perfectly. Lorraine, who I hardly know, is pleasantly correct. Barbara's Mediterranean hand is lifeless even as her expressive, dark, face is animatedly attempting to conceal her feelings. Hanna gives me a strong grip, and in response to my thanks, she tells me, in her guttural gritty tone, that she was just doing her job. Angela looks at my outstretched hand with disdain. "Get over here," she commands, and envelops me in her busom. "Martin is going to be all right and we'll take care of him till he is."

Marty is impatiently waiting for me. He is sitting as tall in his bed as I've seen him, like an animal keenly peering through the underbrush. When we see each other we immediately give up the pretense. I cry a little. I tell him I am not crying over his condition. Feigning somewhat myself, I tell him I am genuinely encouraged and believe he is on his way toward recovery. I tell him I cry because I won't see him for a while.

I am molten inside. My heart aches and flutters. We embrace through the plastic awkwardly, finally planting our lips together on opposite sides of the curtain. Words are choking in our throats. I back out of the immediate area and sit in a chair in the corridor to remove my booties for the last time. Marty sits up high in bed, watching. He waves. I wave. We blow kisses. He puts his fist in the air, triumphantly. I close the heavy door behind me and unleash the flood. Sobbing, I duck into the nearby waiting room and give full vent to my feelings. Minutes later, composed, I blot my eyes all the way to the elevator, heedless of the stares.

I am determined that the rest of the day should go smoothly, without incident, leaving me little time to dwell on sadness. I try to expunge Marty from my immediate thoughts, at least his vivid image. I fight against confusion, excess of emotion. I force myself to concentrate on the precise route, the time, the mechanics of returning the car, not losing my ticket, being sure of all my belongings. I stop in a designated rest stop along the highway and open the trunk to obsessively inventory my two bags even though I vividly remember putting them in.

I fail to exit at the proper place for the Bronx Whitestone Bridge. I estimate I will lose 15 minutes, easily compensated for in my calculations but giving me an uneasy feeling. I ask an elderly man, dressed in sport clothes, leisurely washing his car, for directions. With measured West Indies speech, attentive to every detail, double checking to make sure of my comprehension, he gives them to me with relish, lavishing more time on the task than I would have wanted him to. His directions are perfect. I regain my way without a hitch, return the rental car, board the plane and fall into a dead sleep, waking as the plane touches down in Cincinnati.

I am exhausted, leaden. I ache. I am weak. My voice is weak. I try to concentrate only on the present, on the immediate.

Arline and Jonathan meet my plane. Their eyes tell how bad I look. Jonathan solicitously insists on retrieving my suitcase and carrying it to his car. I don't protest. I feel relieved when we clear the airport and head toward his house. I slump heavily into the seat. The green, northern Kentucky countryside excites me, the billboards flying past the car ratchet my spirits upward. I feel liberated. The conversation in the car and the noise of the motor and the moist air rushing in through open window confirms that I am alive, that possibilities remain available to me, that soon I will hold my first grandchild. For the moment little Asa's face, known to me only from photographs, is in my mind, not Marty's.

The slamming of the front door startles the one month old Asa out of his milk stupor. Diane had finished nursing him minutes before and he had not yet fallen asleep in her arms. He makes small sounds, not of annoyance or demand, just curious, lung-exercising sounds. He flails his hands, articulating at the wrists and cranes his head in a seemingly random fashion, tracking me with his gaze. I put my bag down quietly and carefully kneel near their chair. Diane smiles an open-faced, defenseless, richly expressive smile at me, a smile of sympathy bordering on condolence, of welcome, of love, of pride in the treasure she was holding. I kiss her softly, continuing our silent conversation. Arline and Jonathan stand close by, watching, happy to live in this moment. The late afternoon sun, dappled by the elm tree dominating the sidewalk in front of the house, streams in through the large street window. We all watch Asa, the residue of his mother's milk lightly crusting his still segmented lips, stretching his arms and legs, twisting his face into a variety of expressions. Asa ruptures the mood with a loud belch. The laugh that follows frightens him and he begins to cry.

I ask to hold him and Diane bids me sit in a nearby chair while Jonathan lowers him to my arms. I touch and stroke his body and kiss his head and hands. Asa looks at me intently, trying to focus on this new creature, strange to his small environment. He studies me carefully, surveying my face in small segments. I feel his weight and his warmth and the generations of the weight and warmth of blood ties between grandfathers and their grandchildren and I am glad that I will have years before me to watch him grow and know him. As I hand him to Jonathan I wonder bleakly about Marty's chances to experience the same.

Marty remains in his plastic isolation while I, unimpeded by illness, am free to travel the world, unthreatened by death. We have reunited, joined as twins once again, and then, once again, we have separated. We have had our chance again, for a moment, forced upon us to be sure, to be as close now, at age 59, as we were as children. We will probably never experience this feeling again. I can't imagine feeling this pain of parting ever again. I think we have run our course as twins, that this last month has been a preparation for the last moment of our twinship, when death comes to us.

It will be desperately hard for the survivor when one of us dies, something I never thought about till recently. Now, prompted by advancing age and Marty's brushes with death the last several years, I have been forced to think about it. I believe the time I spent with Marty during the transplant has made it clear to me why it will be so hard.

For non twins the death of even the most beloved person is the death of another. For Marty and me there is no entirely discrete other. There is still a part of each of us that has not completely differentiated from the other. A part we share. Probably a small part, after all the years of being apart and living different lives. And that part will die in the surviving twin, not as a cheap poetic, not as a simile, but an actual deadening of some fraction of the living organism, some part of the will or the spirit or the mind or the body. That partial death of the surviving twin will leave him with the worst of all worlds: the fearful experience of death and the grief of the mourner for both his brother and for himself.

AFTER

Marty was able to leave the hospital about two weeks after I left him in New Haven. The transplant was a success. My marrow was colonizing in his body, his counts were all acceptable, he was afebrile, and he had convinced the doctors that his appetite was returning. He was also weak, dispirited and in considerable pain. Although thankful for having survived the transplant, he was fearful about being away from immediate medical attention.

He was given careful, detailed instructions about how to conduct his life during his convalescence. Among those instructions were several mimeographed pages called, "Discharge Diet Guidelines For Individuals After Bone Marrow Transplantation." The guidelines were meant to sound like helpful household hints and perky suggestions from the Sunday newspaper. With headings that read "Foods to Enjoy at Discharge" and "More Foods to Enjoy at 60 Days From Discharge" and "Never," it became clear just how dangerous the next months would be. His immune system was as fragile as a new born baby's and, after what he had just been through, it was housed in a prematurely old and sick body. When he grew stronger he would receive inoculations against childhood illnesses. The threat of infection, lurking everywhere in the contaminated world he was preparing to rejoin, added anxiety to his ever-present back and midsection pain and profound fatigue. Marty was alive, if not exactly well.

The early winter closed Marty down, depressed him more than he had been in the tiny laminar flow room he had just left. He had more freedom of movement at home but he could not avail himself of that freedom. It was too cold to go outside and his undiagnosed back and stomach pain kept him hunched over when he walked. Worse than that, it prevented him from exercising, something he longed for during his confinement and which he was determined to do to regain his muscle tone. He developed shingles, a painful and not uncommon consequence of his ordeal. He dragged himself around the house, in doubt as to whether he would ever recover. Being alive and remaining in that pitiable state was not what he had bargained for. I went to see him in early November.

The look in Vilunya's face told me much. Her frightened and bewildered eyes beckoned me to a private, conspiratorial conversation sometime during my visit. She needed an ally. Marty approached from the other room. He was swathed in layers of clothes: sweatpants, sweatshirt over layers of other shirts, a small, beautiful alpaca blanket draped over his shoulder, a baseball cap with a silly saying. Slightly bent, he raised his head to look at me. His cadaverous face broke into a crooked smile and acknowledged with a raised eyebrow that he was glad to see me and apologetic for his low state. He extended his arms brittly, letting me know the embrace should not be a forceful one.

"Let me go and wash myself to get the germs from the plane off me." They watched me while I went to the bathroom silently cursing myself for raising the subject of danger to his health before I even settled in. Washed, I joined them in the kitchen. They were both smiling. A bottle of Marty's favorite rum was on the table. There was only one glass.

"Have a belt?"

"Can you drink?"

"Probably, in moderation, although I don't have the taste for it. I'll enjoy watching you."

"Nah, I'd better not. I still feel the drink I had on the plane. Any more right now and I'll get sloshed." I looked from one of them to the other. "How're you doing?"

Neither one answered me. Both Vilunya and Marty looked at each other, at me, at the table. Their struggle to maintain neutral expressions answered sufficiently. I waited. Finally, I said, "It's been hard, huh?"

Marty shifted in his seat. With his fingers he distractedly explored beneath the sleeve of his sweatshirt, exposing the beginning of the black mark left by the numerous hematomas he had suffered. His forearm, with the blackened remnants of collapsed superficial veins looked like that of a drug addict. "Yeah. It shouldn't have been a surprise. By now we all should have been adept at understanding the medical euphemisms. I didn't think there would be all this pain and debility."

"How is your energy, your strength?"

"Nil. It's all I can do to drag myself around. Most of the day I flake out on the couch. I can't seem to get warm enough. I build a big fire and make it too hot for anyone else. I just lay there and rot. I watch any kind of crap on the television."

Vilunya, her hands folded tightly in front of her, her face wrinkled in concentration, a student at attention, said, in an effort to temper the moment, "Yesterday was a lousy day. We had to go to the doctor. Martin's catheter, the Hickman, the one in the chest, needed to be repaired. There's always the worry of infection when they fool around with the catheter. They kept us waiting a long time. The procedure hurt Martin. He had to wear a face mask. He hates it." She took his hand consolingly.

Marty acknowledged the truth of Vilunya's last statement with a sour, averted, look. "At least they confirmed that I do have shingles. I'm sick of having these undiagnosed maladies. The doctors only seem concerned with symptoms they can measure, like blood counts, electrical impulses, lines on X-rays." I fidgeted in my chair, starting to speak. "I know, I know," Marty said preemptively, "It's only been two months."

"Less than two months, a week less," I interrupted.

"Yeah, well, whatever, I know that it's not enough time to see results. I'm just impatient. It seems like I've been a wreck for a year now. I'm just a little sick of it."

We all sat in the strained quiet. There was nothing anyone could have said at that moment that would not have sounded foolish or Pollyanish.

Marty lightly slapped his hands, with spread fingers, on the table. His face opened with a forced smile. "Okay, that's enough of whining and complaining and *kvetching*. Sauly's here and we're going to have a good time, right?" He looked with mock sternness, first at me and then at Vilunya, holding his gaze until he drew a smile. "Now, you, Saul, pour yourself a drink."

I did. We sat and exchanged questions and answers about our children and Asa. After a while Marty asked to be excused. He said he was feeling tired and wanted to lie down on the couch for a while. He insisted that Vilunya and I continue visiting. He lumbered into the living room where I was sure he was going to watch one of his favorite news programs.

Vilunya waited until Marty turned on the television set at the high volume his diminished hearing required.

"I'm glad you came. It's been rough around here. I keep trying to get him to do some light exercise and he keeps resisting. You know your brother. His body may be weak now but his will is still as strong as iron."

"Do you think he can do more right now?"

"I don't know. When I try to push him he gets surly. He tells me that he will know when the time is right to do more and that he'll do it then. I'm a little afraid to press any more."

"Maybe I can help. The worst that will happen is that he'll tell me to kiss his ass and he's told me that before. What do think it is he can do?"

"That's the hard part. Real exercise is out of the question for the time being. Maybe helping him, or rather, encouraging him first and then helping him, to clean up his study. He's been talking about it but not doing it."

Vilunya began preparing dinner and I walked into the living room to join Marty. He was asleep, breathing noisily, his head at an awkward angle. Someone on McNeil-Lehrer with a Slavic accent was making an overly sincere argument about our policy toward Bosnia. I turned the set off and looked at Marty asleep, crumpled on the couch. He uttered a child's sleep sigh, a wistful, sadness-tinged sound, a plea for relief not forthcoming.

"Vilunya tells me you want to clean up your study. Want me to help you? We could build a fire in the stove and get the room toasty. I could do the heavy work."

Marty eyed me appraisingly. He shifted his weight on the couch, making himself more comfortable, not preparing to rise. "There's nothing that needs doing in there that can't wait until I'm completely up to it. You're not here to perform domestic chores for me."

"It's not a domestic chore. It's something that you want to do and I'd be glad to help you with it. I think it will engage you, maybe break your routine a little. Besides, we'll be together, visiting. What do you say?" I put enough emphasis into my words so that Marty knew it wasn't an argument I intended to lose; that, for the moment, I wouldn't allow his weakness to be a shield.

"I really don't feel strong enough right now to give it a real effort. Why don't you sit down here and relax."

"Look, if you don't feel up to going into the study, just tell me what shelves you want to work on. I'll bring the stuff in here and you can look at it and decide what stays and what goes. I want to be of some help to you, and I've been here a day just sitting and eating. It'll give me something to do, too."

Marty looked directly at me. His look was not entirely friendly. He knew as well as I did what we would be embarking upon and, although he didn't like it, he felt trapped by my argument. "Okay, but until I tell you I've had it, okay?" I nodded assent. "There is a bookcase on the back wall that has some cardboard files labeled LASA on a shelf near the top. Start with those. If you could bring in a handful I can tell what should stay and what should go."

We worked for thirty or forty minutes. As Marty decided what he would keep I replaced those things in the empty space in the bookcase. The items to be discarded, mostly loose paper, I tossed into a pile on the floor, on the side of the fireplace. Marty started to fidget.

"What are you going to do with the pile of trash?"

"Can I burn it in the fireplace?"

"Not that much. It's too messy. The blackened paper residue will get into the room and a lot will be left in the fireplace to clean."

"I'll pack it into a trash bag and put it out with the garbage for pickup."

"Yeah, I guess you'll have to. Well, listen, thanks for the help," he said with a false lightness. "Maybe tomorrow we could do some more if we're both up for it."

"How about more right now? You look like you have the energy for a little more work."

Marty's face turned dark and hot. With some effort he sat up on the couch. "What the hell are you thinking, that I'm malingering, that it's my idea of fun to sit here like a slug, that I like doing nothing? Don't you understand that I do all I can possibly do. I know you want to help but you'll just have to take my word for it that I'm at the end of my energy right now." He remained poised, demanding an answer from me.

"I do believe you, Marty, " I said in a somewhat chastened but unapologetic voice. "Just pushing you a little. It's your job to get better. It's my job to push. Between us we don't have to be subtle, do we?"

Marty sized up the last remark. His face softened slightly. "Do your job better or I'll fire you. Now get into the kitchen and pour yourself a drink and come back in here and sit down."

"Okay, boss, I be back soon." Before I turned to leave Marty and I contested to see who would be the first to reveal the smile behind the mask.

Marty called me in January. His words held a current of expectancy.

He had something to tell me, something that would come later in the conversation, in his own time. We waded through the perfunctory, but necessary, clearing of the underbrush of potentially fearsome facts. No, he wasn't feeling worse, no fevers, no extraordinary pain, no feelings of depression. The weather was intermittently bitterly cold or snowing heavily. His diet continued to bore him. He wanted more spice, more taste. And yet, though no fact that he had recited showed any change in his environment, I could hear lightness in his account. Out with it!

"I can't explain it completely, but I'm getting my body back."

"Hey, hey, that's great!" I didn't exactly know what he meant, and I almost regretted my cry of joy, but I knew that his wasn't a spur of the moment crack. "Tell me, tell me."

"Probably about a week ago I began to feel something alive in my body. A sinew, a muscle, a little snap to a reflex, things that I haven't felt in a year. It has been just about a year that I have been sinking and just these last days I feel like I am rising. For a few days now I have been trying to do the Kabat-Zinn body scan. Just today I got through the whole thing. It would be hard to say what good it did but getting through it without having to interrupt it in agony made me feel, well, accomplished. Yesterday I read for a while. I just turned the goddamned television set off and read. Not for long, maybe twenty minutes, but I was able to concentrate." Lowering his tone and slowing the pace, he said, "And last night I was able to sleep almost the whole night through without a sleeping pill. I'm telling you, man, my body is coming back to me. I know that it's real." He had burned his passport from the other land. He was back, admitted, stamped, home, for good.

"Oh, Marty, your voice is confirmation. If I wasn't afraid of being struck by lightning I'd say God be praised. God bless you. Welcome."

We exulted in amused silence at my uncharacteristic benediction for a while and then Marty poured out his plans: he would make arrangements to resume teaching next September, he'd continue working on his book about El Salvador, he would enter a regimen of physical therapy and pursue it vigorously, he would practice yoga and meditation, he would help dear Vilunya around the house and stop being bad tempered, he would play the guitar after an absence of years, maybe get a teacher, travel to Arizona to see us before the winter was over, he would live. He would get well. He would live.

Less than two months later Marty was in Arizona for a ten day visit.

He came alone. Vilunya said she could not leave her business for that long. I had the impression she needed a small vacation from Marty. For weeks before his arrival I tried to determine what health precautions should be taken. Arizona and several other desert areas in the southwest is host to a disease called Valley Fever. It is transmitted through a spore found in the ground. Our house is in the desert. Approximately 25 percent of the long time residents have had the disease, many of them without being aware of it, as was the case with Arline, who suffered with it for a year before she was diagnosed. Fatigue is the major symptom, something Marty didn't need more of. It is very seldom fatal but it can inflict damage to the lungs and other parts of a healthy system. Marty was particularly susceptible to any kind of fungal infection. I had to determine the risk to Marty this soon after the transplant. I spoke to local doctors as well as to the Bone Marrow Transplant center at the University of Arizona in Tucson and reported my findings to Marty. It was determined that the risk was low and could be made much lower if Marty wore a face mask. Because I knew that Marty hated the face mask and that he would be tempted to forget his, I stocked up on them and placed them prominently in the room he was to occupy.

He used a mask the first day we walked in the desert but not even my nagging would persuade him to don it from that day on. We walked in the desert almost every day of his visit. He seemed to grow stronger each succeeding day, walking faster and farther. The visit was a great success. My fears for his health were overwhelmed by the evidence of his improved looks and stamina. He had color for the first time in a year. For part of every day Marty sat in the sun happy with his new found freedom of movement, confirming to him that he was not an invalid. He still had abdominal and back pain and he tired easily, but he walked through his pain and he snoozed whenever he felt drowsy. There were no tears when he left. We were all certain that his recovery was well on its way.

Carol and Ray and Pon, Marty's fellow patients in the Unit, did not do as well. Pon was brought back to the hospital with an infection that his compromised immune system could not resist, and there he died. Ray and Carol never left the Unit. Both were overwhelmed by their disease and the side effects of the transplant. I could not help but think of what the death of three out of the four patients in the Unit did to Marylou's statistics.

I proposed a *vuelva de vida* (return of life) trip through northern New Mexico for just Marty and me. He had resumed teaching in the fall of

1994. After negotiating the time off several weeks after school started, he agreed. He had improved all through the late winter and spring. On August 22nd he had a triumphant birthday party. I was tempted to go but it seemed like a lot of travel and expense for an essentially frivolous purpose. Besides, deep in my mind was the thought that I still might have to make emergency trips to see Marty.

We met in Albuquerque late in the evening, almost a year to the day after his discharge from the unit. Marty's hair had grown completely back, somewhat curly at the edges and as black as ever. He still moved tentatively but his color was good and he had filled out a little. Tired from his trip all he wanted was a snack and bed. We set out the next morning at a pace I determined would not be too demanding. There were no mishaps. Nothing spoiled a minute of it, not the weather, not a cabin I had booked that turned out to be a shack crowded by other shacks, not the waitresses in Dulce, cackling in a mixture of high plains Texas and Spanish over the oddity of the old twins. We were sad when we parted only because we hated for it to end but confident there would be more trips like it.

Marty caught a six pound rainbow on the San Juan River. Immediately after the camera clicked the commemorative snapshot with the fish, he slumped slightly against the gunwale of the boat, a sad shadow dimming the light across his smiling face. He caught my eye, sorry that I had seen his expression. We both knew in that precise moment that his full strength and vigor would never return; that he would have to settle for what was left to him.

September 22, 1994
Mano,

The involuntary movie projector in my mind keeps replaying scenes of our trip. Every time I decide to tarry over a particularly delicious moment it gets replaced with one even more vivid and sweet in the memory.

One moment I'm standing at the pond at the Oso Lodge looking north at the mountains rising into Colorado and the next we're driving through the narrow river valley northeast of Cuba where we polished off a fiery adobado and heading toward Coyote, or standing in the clean, wood-smelling room of the Tierra Wool Company watching the strong women standing near their looms, or looking at the all but abandoned courthouse in Tierra Amarilla where Reyes Tijerina and his men killed the two marshals, or feeling the flutter of excitement coming down the grade from the Navajo Dam to the San Juan, or having that hog on my line and wondering whether I'd get him close enough to the boat for Johnny to net before my wrist fell off, or sitting in Mr. Trujillo's meager living room looking through his wet flies, or feeling the slight flush of familiarity with the country returning to Chama through the Jicarillo reservation. Many other thoughts and scenes of fleeting encounters with people and observations of the landscape flood my mind.

But what came back to me most of all was being with you and schliedering and schlondering through northern New Mexico, drinking beer and whiskey, laughing at manic jokes that, if overheard by normal people, would make us candidates for the rubber room, singing heroic songs of Mexican heroes and their horses and talking, just talking, of everything, of our children, our wives, of Dad. It was a great joy to celebrate the first anniversary of your rebirth It put to rest doubts and dark thoughts that have been with me for a long time.

All my senses gave me the proof that you are indeed back. You may have a way to go to regain all your physical strength, but the eye hungry for new sights, the mind eager for new ideas, those are fully back and the rest will surely follow.

Welcome back, my dear brother, with all my heart, welcome back.
Saul

Marty returned to teaching and the full range of academic activity with more relish than I'd ever remembered him having in his healthy years. Perhaps it was to compensate for his unvoiced belief that it would be a long time, if ever, before he could go to the field. He plunged into his work, resumed writing his book on El Salvador and energetically engaged in academic debate. If he was diminished physically, he could still be strong intellectually. He took particular delight in the careers of some of his younger colleagues, praising their work, always speaking highly of them. He felt pleased that the discipline he had served all his life was in their hands.

Marty read an article in a Latin American journal that enraged him. He thought the conclusions wrong and the scholarship faulty. He weighed into the debate with a thirty page paper, attacking the offending work. We talked about it on the phone many times. He sent me a draft of his paper. The subject at issue never engaged me but what was exciting for me to observe was the feeling it aroused in Marty. He was at war. Compared to the battle he had waged for the last year-and-a-half the stakes in this contest were trivial but he attacked with abandon. Look out, I thought, with a twinge of sympathy for his adversary, Marty's back.

His health was improving slowly, but not without setbacks. In the middle of the school year he developed low grade fevers, which robbed him of energy and depressed him. His mind conjured the worst. He became less communicative. He shortened our phone conversations and was somewhat remote during them.

January 14, 1995
Mano,

I've been thinking of you more than usual since you developed the fevers that have been plaguing you the past couple of weeks. It made me realize that my thoughts of you occur less often as you get healthier. It has been some time since those thoughts had the character of a vigil.

In the middle of this letter I look out the window at a sky full of clouds of many colors and shapes, a rarity in Phoenix. We had a drenching rain last night and everything feels cold and fresh and vigorous today. A hawk is flying close enough to my fifth floor window so that I can see the occasional flapping feather. His dark body is so clearly contrasted with the brilliantly white background of the clouds that he appears closer than I know him to be. He is flying away from me quickly. Even though he is getting smaller he is plainly visible because of his swooping movements. Finally, at what appears from my window to be the other side of Squaw Peak, close perhaps to where we live, he becomes a dot and vanishes. I have a small pang as I straighten in my chair to finish the letter. That is how I know that hawk-watching is my form of solitaire playing, a flight from labor, from doing or thinking about the difficult. In this case, not wanting to think about you're being sick.

This time, however, it's somewhat different. I don't have the dark thoughts about you that have been with me for the last few years. I am confident that your present ailment is temporary and something that your system will fight off. My belief doesn't come from science. Lang and Kettyle will give you that. Mine comes from witchcraft and Corsicanism! And also from, I regret to say, my own feelings of age ambushing me. I won't reel off the list of symptoms. You are well aware of them and of the variations peculiar to your own body.

I'm sure I can't fully understand the blackness that comes over you when you get sick, particularly at a time like this when you seem to be roaring back to full health. It never gives you proper warning. It must always produce doubts in your mind. If you can do it, try to think of the tremendous gains you have made till now. If you charted those gains and the occasional setback, it seems to me, the setbacks, of which this is one, would look like small blips, hardly interfering with the upward trajectory.

For my part dear bruderl, I am conceding certain things to age. I am trying to slow certain things in my life, and trying to change activities and behaviors that wear me out with anxiety. I am thinking of what life will be like and what I will do when I end my active business life. The more I think about it the less afraid I am of it. I also find I can accomplish the same without driving myself. And that gives me more time to watch hawks.

I hope you can do the same and that you'll feel better soon.

Un abrazo,

Saul

For the next year Marty lived his life almost as fully as before the transplant. His health improved sufficiently so that it ceased being a daily concern. During that time he even had a cold that responded well to antibiotics and his own defenses. He maintained his teaching and writing, visited close-by friends, had dinners in restaurants, traveled a little and went sailing several times. With the exception of the full return of his physical strength he was back.

Marty and Vilunya visited us in Phoenix in April, 1996, during our truncated version of spring. The desert wildflowers were in bloom and so was Marty. We were all in high spirits, propelled by Marty's undeniable return to health. We spent a day at an arboretum east of Phoenix. On the way, in the car, Marty and I let what had begun as a dry discussion of welfare legislation erupt into an extended argument. Forced by a construction job on the highway to wait twenty or thirty minutes, we went at each other with an intensity we hadn't allowed in discussions like these for many years. We gave each other hell. Arline and Vilunya considered us both crazy. It left no residue of bad feeling. We walked for miles in the arboretum, slowly, observing the fantastic array of plants collected from all over the world, talking as we walked, finishing with a lavish picnic. As I walked with Vilunya I speculated cheerfully that Marty appeared 85 percent restored. She hesitantly told me that 75 percent was closer.

The visit was full of activity: eating, drinking, laughter. Marty's life was good and getting better. Aaron would graduate from college in a couple of months and Leah would marry in the summer. For me, something was almost settled. Inwardly, I used the word cured for the first time.

Marty and Vilunya left Phoenix for Los Angeles to visit with Mom and Phil before returning to Boston. In Los Angeles, Marty noticed a swelling in his neck, which in the time it took to return home, grew to the size of a large egg. Lengthy tests confirmed lymphoma, probably the converted residue of the CLL cells not killed in preparation for the transplant two-and-a-half years prior.

More chemotherapy, more radiation, more recovery. In the language of medical euphemism, the results were satisfactory. The tumor was shrunk. The cost was debilitating fatigue, a general weakening and moments of despair. Vilunya gave up her business. She made no declarations at the time, nothing about needing the time to care for Marty. She simply said she had been in business for many years and it was now time to do other things. It was obvious, though, that the latest health setback unnerved her. She didn't have the strength for both business and Marty.

Marty, Vilunya and Leah went to Aaron's graduation in upstate New York. The family picture taken then shows a beaming Marty, grateful at being present at the important family milestone. In preparation for Leah and Tom's August wedding Marty suspended chemotherapy. He appeared, resplendently dressed, a large Panama hat covering his again bald head and shading his steroid swollen face. The speech he made from the wedding canopy to Leah and Tom, in the clear and strong voice though it was, was made all the more poignant by the state of his health.

The chemotherapy was working. Marty continued teaching in the fall. The trend was good we were told. Remissions are easy to achieve with lymphoma and if the time between relapses is great enough, so the implied reasoning seemed to go, well, it's all a time game anyway, isn't it? The worst was that lymphoma plunged Marty, as well as the rest of us, back into the medical miasma we thought we had been extricated from. Marty had numerous appointments with doctors, almost always accompanied now by Vilunya. They would receive answers they couldn't quite be sure of, forecasts a little too vague. Vilunya researched herbal medicines, dietary aids, vitamin and other medicinal supplements and urged Marty into a regimen of them. He finished the semester, weary and bedraggled, but pleased that he had fulfilled his obligations at work. He needed the time between semesters to restore his energy.

Early in February his doctor prescribed a series of frequent and aggressive radiation treatments, pinpointed at the remains of the tumor, to kill it root and branch. The radiation lasted almost a month.

Email
March 17, 1997
Yo, tzololishke:

Mon. afternoon, finished teaching. All I have to do is complete the paper I'm giving tomorrow at noon at Harvard. It's almost done and the thought that someone published exactly what I will say (only better) has entered my mind but flown away quickly. I think I've got the goods but if not I'll deny that anyone else has a valid critique of my work.

The effect of radiation seems to come and go. Yesterday I was a wreck and today I feel stronger. It appears that after several days of it I go down. Thank god this is the last week. The doc said that I might need some extra treatments that will be less harmful. I think I'll learn how they make that decision tomorrow when I see him. Being depleted of energy is the worst thing that can happen because it also robs me of hope. I fill with fantasies of death and almost welcome it. I know it will improve and Vilunya, the darling, is full of encouragement and soothing words. She suffers greatly yet still remains hopeful and bright. She realizes that I will never regain my previous health and still has not thrown me overboard.

If this Friday is the last treatment, next week is Spring break and I hope I can shuck all the effects during that time. We may go to New Hampshire again, hopefully this time to walk and move more than before. Or to sit and look at the lake from the inside. Either way.

It was good to see Aaron this weekend. He's really coming along and sounds more realistic about many things.

Going home now for a nap.

Love,
Marty

Email
Feb. 17, 1997
Dear Marty,

I hope when you read this you'll be on your way to give your lecture, books under arm, coat flying in a self-created breeze, feeling refreshed and full of energy. Short of that, just appearing for your lecture will be a considerable victory.

You once asked me, only partially rhetorically, I believe, what the various medical people meant when they said they wanted patients who were fighters. You are one of the last people of all who need an explanation. You are too busy fighting to dwell on how it looks to be fighting. I admire your plan to teach today and tomorrow and to incorporate the radiation into your normal daily activities.

Keep fighting. Never give up. Never! Never! Fighting is healthy. Fighting is curative. Luchando matará el pinche cancerito.

Love,

Saul

Email

Feb. 18, 1997

Thank you for that lovely message yesterday. My kind of fighting is called schlepping. I'll schlep until I fall down. And then I'll start rastreando or some other form of movement or lack of movement. You can take that to the bank.

My routine yesterday and today has been not unlike last semester. I'm usually invigorated by class and exhausted afterward. The invigoration is worth the other. I've slowly begun yoga and think it will do me good but getting around is a bit of a problem. Tomorrow the radiation begins again. I'll schlep through that. Talk to you soon.

Martin

The doctors felt the results were excellent. A gallium scan showed no trace of the lymphoma, although a CTscan showed fluid in his lungs. That presented a problem. Marty had decided that he was going to the Latin American Studies Association convention in Guadalajara, Mexico in April.

"Do you think it's prudent to go to Mexico right now?"

"I don't know, but it's been three-and-a-half years since the transplant and I've not been in Latin America once. This seems like the perfect time and place. I'll see LASA colleagues that I haven't seen or talked to in years."

"Are you feeling strong enough?"

Marty laughed a quiet, deep, ironic laugh. "I don't know when I'm going to feel any stronger. And whether I go or not will depend to some degree on the results of the CTscan or chest X-ray, or whatever the hell they are going to give me in a few days to determine whether there still is fluid in my lungs. If I go, I'll take it easy. I'll be rooming with Jack Spence. If I get into trouble I can rely on Jack to help me"

A couple of days before the trip Marty called to tell me that the X-ray showed very little fluid. His doctor approved the trip, and armed him with diuretics and antibiotics. I wished him a good trip. After we hung up I stared out of my office window, out across the Phoenix Indian School campus to Camelback Mountain and the sky beyond and imagined what his trip would be like. I thought I heard a certain resignation in his voice over the last several weeks as we discussed the trip. I thought I heard the voice of our family, of those living, including me, and of those dead: Dad and his people, most of whom we never knew, people to whom sorrow and death was as natural as life. Marty did not want to die. Neither did he want to live if it meant sitting in a cold sun, a blanket over a worn out and useless body, waiting for someone to come and wipe the drool from his chin. If the trip to Mexico would be too much for him, he would die there. Not a bad place for Marty to die, a place he loved.

I thought that unceremonious, brief conversation was the last I would ever have with Marty; that he would die in Mexico, that I would never see him again. It was a thought, a premonition, but so strong it immediately began to insert itself in my mind as a fact. I recited the thought quickly to myself, not wanting to dwell on it at length. Over the next few days I waited for the phone call to confirm my worst fears. It almost happened.

Marty was hospitalized in Mexico with what was ultimately diagnosed as congestive heart failure. He was stabilized there and put on a plane for home. During the flight he needed oxygen. He thought a day or two of rest would restore him. In a couple of days he was in Mount Auburn hospital receiving oxygen and a variety of medications. Vilunya told me later that she thought he was dying until they gave him a heart stimulant and he started improving immediately.

Shortly after I arrived at the hospital, a few days after he was admitted, Marty removed his oxygen mask, declaring that he no longer needed it. His breathing was shallow and labored. His eyes were piercing, his expression fixed in concentration. He was trying to assess his body's reaction to the damage his heart had suffered. The doctors agreed that his heart failure was caused by the Adryamiacin he had taken in several of his chemotherapies. The drug had damaged his heart muscle, severely and irreversibly. He could be stabilized, but substantial improvement was impossible. Marty didn't ask the doctors for a prognosis. He would find the answer himself. Vilunya was forecasting his recovery, treating this latest insult as an episode, something that medication and exercise would remedy. Perhaps not a complete recovery, but certainly a vast improvement. If he was having them, Marty did not want to communicate his bleak thoughts to

Vilunya. Her strength came from feelings of optimism fueled by dread of the alternative. She would need all her strength.

In the short, slow, walks we took in the hospital corridor, he held either Vilunya or me tightly by the arm and rested once before returning to his bed, exhausted. We sat in silence during one of those walks, just the two of us. We kept exchanging heavy glances. Marty had something to tell me. I said nothing. I waited.

"I think there's a chance I can improve somewhat as soon as they stabilize the medicines. At least enough to be able to drive, slowly go up and down the stairs to my office, work on my book."

"Don't decide yet. Maybe more improvement than that is possible. You've been defying medical predictions right along."

"Yeah, maybe, we'll see," he said sourly. "I can live with this blow, as long as I don't become a burden. What I don't think I have the strength to fight anymore is another round of leukemia if it returns." We looked each other full in the eyes for a while, without speaking.

I thought Marty was raising the subject to implant the thought in me of helping him to die should his worst fears be realized. I could have been wrong. I thought it was the wrong time to have a conversation about death so I didn't ask him to elaborate. I knew I would do it if he asked. I had helped Dad to die without ever having any regret. As the thought of hastening Marty's death began to take shape a terror seared through my consciousness. Even without fleshing out the thought, without seeing the place where it would happen, what method would be employed or what the emotional tone would be, I knew that rather than an act performed on behalf of someone else, for me it would be an act of suicide.

After a several week hospitalization Marty returned home, weakened, further impaired, to resume life. He accepted what had happened to him with grace and determinedly sought to make good use of what was left to him. He progressed, able to increase his activity more than I, and I am sure, the doctors I had consulted, thought possible. Although he moved slowly and his breathing was labored, he drove himself to his office and worked on his book. He talked about the book constantly. It became a talisman. He would not die until the book was finished. He accepted his diminished state without complaint. It was the end of May, planting time, and Marty found things to enjoy.

The man who greeted me in his office as I arrived for our appointment told me, as we were shaking hands, that my secretary had called ahead and asked me to call her. When I reached her she told me that Vilunya had called and her voice sounded urgent. I refused the proffered phone in the small, close office. Instead I went outside, found some shade and called Vilunya on a cellular phone.

"I hope you're sitting down," she said. Wryly, I noted the spines and thorns on all the plants around me and the sharp decorative gravel ground cover as I waited in silence for what would follow. "Martin's counts have gone crazy. Five days ago his white count was seven to eight thousand. Today it is one hundred thirteen thousand. They believe it is an acute form now."

"Does it mean what it sounds like?"

"The doctors think so. From an enzyme test they think there may be some liver damage. They'll do more tests tomorrow to learn more, but they are both talking of end stage treatments." Her voice rasped over the words "end stage" as she struggled to maintain composure. Now was not the time to let loose, the resolve in her voice signaled.

"How is Marty?"

"Weak and sad. He's resting now, but he wanted me to call you right away. He'll speak to you a little later. Aaron knows because he went with us to the doctor. Leah and Tom are coming to dinner tonight. We'll discuss his death with them." We both let silence soothe the moment. Questions started forming in my mind.

"What does end stage treatments mean? Have the doctors made any time predictions?"

"Mostly experimental techniques, clinical trials, methods not yet approved. We're going to do a search to see if there is any program he can get into. His hematologist, Lange, says it's between weeks and months. He says he's going to give him a drug called Vincristine. It would be a palliative, something to lower the counts a little. A full course of chemotherapy would kill him now."

"What does Kettyle say?" Dr. Kettyle, Marty's health plan doctor, a righteous, steady-eyed, slow talking man, had promised them complete honesty.

"You know, he's not a hematologist, but he believes it is the end. His face had the look of doom."

Marty and Vilunya began putting his affairs in order, making preparations for his death, an updated will, medical directive, retirement from teaching and arrangements for his pension.

245

Marty asked certain people to visit him, to say goodbye. In early June, I met Phil and Mom in Lexington. A few friends of theirs were there also. We all knew, or knew of, each other. Visiting in small groups or, all together during lengthy meals, we wove a fabric of Marty's life of people who represented different eras and relationships. The mood was by no means unrelievedly sad. We cried together, the three brothers, Vilunya and Mom. We also laughed and talked of the days of our childhood, of our marriages and children, of Dad, of better times. There was very little explicit talk of death. Marty repeated, when appropriate, the clinical facts like a scientist. Mom, approaching her eighty-seventh year, her recently broken ankle in a cast, kept talking of a miracle. Before she left she declared that she would return August 22nd to celebrate our birthday with Marty and Vilunya.

And then, as if responding both to the treatment and Mom's plea, the counts started reversing. Within weeks the white count went from 280,000 to 44,000. And, strangest of all, almost no sign of the blasts, or the acute form, were present. What remained was the CLL, the disease he had started with, and, by all accounts, more manageable than the acute form. Good news. A reprieve. From chronic to acute is the usual progression. From acute to chronic is unheard of. According to Dr. Lange, nothing in the literature could be found to explain it. He said he saw a similar case in 1978 in a patient who lives to this day.

Marty reached me in California, where Arline and I were visiting with our daughter Bess and her family, to tell me of this marvel. His voice was shaky and weak. "Lange suspended the Vincristine because the counts are so good. I'm depleted of platelets. They've given me a transfusion and I'll get another in a day or so." His voice was low, attempting unsuccessfully to keep his tone clinical, informative.

"That's good news, the acute form going away," I said carefully, tentatively. I was worried at the way he sounded and confused at what he was telling me. "How is all this hitting you? Or would you rather answer in a few days when I see you?"

"A few weeks ago I was preparing for death. Now, that seems to be put off, for how long I don't know. I don't know what to make of it. I need to get a little stronger before I can understand it." His voice broke. He began crying. "I can't talk any more. I'll see you soon."

Vilunya met Arline and me at the terminal exit, her face bright with smiles. Marty was sitting behind the wheel of the car parked at the curb, waiting. We talked happily, though somewhat nervously, of what we would do in the following days; where we would have dinner, the planned overnight trip to New Hampshire. Although Marty moved slowly, unsteadily, he was alert and engaged. The visit unfolded in an atmosphere of subdued normalcy, exchanging detailed news of children, family gossip, broadening to news and gossip of a wider group.

Marty was making good progress on his book. He had enlisted friends to help in research and editing. He told me he was confident he would live at least until the end of summer. We spent hours going through his collection of recordings to find a certain piece of music he wanted played at his memorial – a *son jarocho*. This stringed music of Vera Cruz, which Marty loved since he first heard it visiting Mexico as a student. Its furious and percussive rhythms, led by the unique harp of the region, would be the sound of remembrance for those who gather to bid him farewell. We couldn't find the exact recording he was looking for but the time spent playing parts of many recordings of jarocho *conjuntos* passed pleasantly, not sadly.

The next day, walking out of doors, Marty stumbled and began falling heavily, barely able to control his movements. I caught him and lowered him gently so he could sit and rest for a moment. He felt like a doll in my arms. He weighed nothing. Marty made light of the incident, but I could tell from the distracted look he had most of the time and his fast diminishing control over his body that the end was sooner than the doctors would say. I wanted to press him to me as we walked or carry him in my arms. I did neither. We were in the midst of ostensibly good news about Marty's condition. I was sure that Marty's body told him differently but he didn't want everyone to dwell on his self-arrived-at sad prognosis. He would live until his last breath.

At the festive dinner before Arline and I left, Vilunya suggested that we return for our birthday, in a little over a month. I contemplated it, mentally rationing trips for medical emergencies I felt certain were looming. I told them it was highly unlikely. Later, in bed, Arline, certain that I wanted to go but anxious about the time and money, suggested it would be a good goal for Marty. As we were leaving we told them we'd come. Pleased by the news, they stood in the doorway holding each other around, waving and smiling sweetly, sadly at us. Every leave-taking, for some time now has had the weight of a final goodbye.

On the first day of August, Vilunya's friend, Sheila, called to tell me that Marty had been taken to Mount Auburn hospital by ambulance with a fever and precipitously low blood pressure, almost unable to move. I asked Sheila for more information, for a prognosis, for conclusions. In a flat, affectless, tone she repeated what she had told me, no more. After several exchanges it came to me that she was telling me only what she knew and she was doing it in such a way as neither to cause me to despair nor to be falsely optimistic. Vilunya was with Marty in the hospital. When I spoke to her an hour later she told me the doctors had told her it was grave. They described his condition as being almost in a coma. They couldn't decide whether it was metabolic or an infection or the lymphoma.

I wasn't interested in their speculations. I knew what it was. It was death calling for Marty. Later in the day, however, he was moved out of the emergency room and into a coronary care unit. All his signs had improved considerably. His trend was up. He was alert. The feeling was that he would, once again, survive, I was told. I went anyway.

Leah and Tom picked me up at the airport and drove me directly to the hospital. As Leah embraced me she told me that Marty was alive and looking much better than he did when he was first admitted. She knew, without my telling her, what thoughts had been rampaging through my mind during the overnight flight.

Marty's eyes followed me as I entered his room and, in the gesture that was now familiar to us, dropped my bag on the way to his bed. He was both happy to see me and apologetic at causing me to make the trip yet again. I threaded my way carefully through the lines attached to his body from the monitoring devices. He closed his eyes with emotion as I stroked and kissed his head. He had a full oxygen mask, not the small nostril tubes he had when he suffered the heart failure. This was worse: two catheters in his heart, one threaded through his neck, the other through his groin, a catheter surgically implanted in his chest that left a large wound.

"The last time you came to my hospital room," Marty said, "I thanked you for coming, and you said to me, 'Where else would I be?'", reminding me and thanking me yet again. He grasped my hand and squeezed it, showing me his strength. His eyes twinkled ironically, and he said, confidently, "Don't worry, *mano*, I've been here before." His voice was muffled through the mask, but strong. We stayed in his room for a couple of hours in distant communication with Marty. We spoke loudly so that he could hear above the sound of the rushing oxygen. He nodded, and from time to time, gave short answers or comments. Although all his signs were good, it looked to me as if his body was surrendering. While Marty slept

I went home with Vilunya to nap, clean up and return in a few hours to have dinner near the hospital and return to Marty's room.

We looked in on Marty before dinner. He seemed slightly agitated. His voice, as he bade us have a nice dinner, had a hard edge. Leah was with him. He took his oxygen mask off, saying he could breathe as well without it. I looked at the monitor. There was no change. Vilunya and I left for dinner.

In the empty lobby of the hospital, on our way to rejoin Marty, the public address system blared a message, unintelligible except for the word, STAT. The sound numbed me, drew me back to the California hospital where Dad lay, facing his end. I said nothing to Vilunya. When we arrived at the Cardiac floor I heard the STAT message repeated. On the way to his room I saw Leah in the visitor's waiting room, trying to talk on the telephone between sobs. She was summoning Aaron, who was performing with his rock band. Marty had gone into cardiac arrest.

The attending doctor explained to us that they had given Marty strong, lifesaving medications and put him on a respirator. He was unconscious, but his signs were strong. The hope was that he would wake up in a short time and be able to breathe without the machine. We sat there like refugees at a hostile border, dumb and frightened. Leah leaned into Tom's chest, feeling his warm strength. Aaron sat on the floor, following the talk with his sad eyes. His somber look told me that he understood all he needed to. Vilunya asked questions to which only the most general and guarded answers were given. She suddenly looked absolutely spent, exhausted beyond her ability to endure. She had to have sleep. Everyone, except me, left to get some sleep and wait for news.

I stayed in the hospital that night. I was certain that Marty would not revive and I didn't want to have to speak to anyone. I tried to make myself comfortable on the undersized plastic couch in the visitor's waiting room. I told myself that I wanted to sleep. My mind would not permit it. I saw Marty in Mexico, lean and brown, pulsing with life, his silky mustache not yet fully grown, squatting near the pottery stall at the market in Tlacolula, speaking to the indigenous merchant. I saw him at the helm of his sailboat, handsome and poised, his posture somewhat theatrical, his shaggy seventies sideburns flying beneath his watch cap. I saw him on Crown Street, giggling uncontrollably as Dad bore down on us in a rage. I saw him in his hospital room, in the intimate embrace of the machine, waiting.

I looked in on him several times that night. His body, activated by the respirator, inflated and collapsed in an awkward, repeated rhythm. On the inbreath an abrupt, almost violent, syncopation. On the exhalation, a desperate quiver. I held his heavy hand, stroked his face and head and talked to him, encouraged him the way I had many times. It sounded false to me. I stopped. Instead I said, "Marty, it's me, Sauly. I'm here with you. Stay with us if you can. But if you can't, you can't." I put my hand lightly on his chest. I rolled his eyelid back to see what flicker of Marty there was. I couldn't find my Marty in that body. Each time I went back to the visitors lounge and tried to curl up on the couch I heard the whisper of the frightened little boy, begging to know, "Where's Marty?"

Early in the morning they came to tell me he had again gone into cardiac arrest and that I should call his wife. Minutes later a team of two doctors and a nurse came to tell me Marty was dead. They surrounded me to catch me if I fell. The young woman doctor took my forearm and told me how sorry she was. Her touch was real. Sorrow at the death of a man and having to tell his mirror image of that death shone through the professional mask.

"Where is he?"

"In his room. Can we get you anything? Would you like to sit down?"

"No. I want to see him."

"It will be a few minutes. We have to do some things."

"Will you come and tell me as soon as I can see him?"

"Yes."

"Thank you."

They left. I washed my face, letting my tears mingle with the cool water. I felt myself strangely alert. Moments later, someone told me I could go into Marty's room. Closing the door behind me, I looked at him carefully, inventorying him. He looked the same to me as the Marty of the night before, except that he wasn't moving in that frighteningly inhuman rhythm of the machine. He was handsome now, no longer entubated, catheterized, respirated, strangled by tubes and wires. He had retired honorably from the field of combat. His expression was confident, dignified. There was no sign of a struggle having been lost. I studied his chest to see if there was any movement, to see if a mistake had been made. No movement. No mistake. A nurse came in, offering me coffee and making sure I had not fainted.

I raised him to an almost upright position to embrace him. He was heavy. His back was wet, the only indication of the life just ended. I lay him down and took his right hand and placed it on my cheek and temple, uncurling his fingers with my hand. Our hands were exactly the same size, our fingernails identical. I kissed his hand and said his name aloud softly, over and over again and wept quietly, feeling myself shrivel and weaken. The twins were gone. I was alone.

We cremated Marty two days later. It took place in a chapel-like room, the oven concealed behind paneled doors. The night before, reminiscing in the kitchen of the house that was no longer Marty and Vilunya's, now just Vilunya's, Leah mentioned, and sang a few words of a song that we all knew Marty had loved. The initial trembling, frightful understanding that Marty was dead had given way to the leaden numbness that, each of us, in our own way, was experiencing. The song was a *son* from the Isthmus of Tehuantepec, the melody and words of which were more wistful than sad, more longing than heroic.

Child, when I die
Don't cry over my tomb
Sing me a beautiful *son, ay mama*
Sing me La Zandunga

Don't cry for me, no, don't cry for me, no
Because if you cry, I die
But if you sing to me
I'll always live and never die.

Margarita Dalton, a friend of Marty and Vilunya's from Oaxaca, in New York on business, came to Lexington with her son, Rodrigo, to comfort Vilunya. Marty was planning to use a poem of her murdered brother, the Salvadoran poet, Roque Dalton, in his book. Margarita agreed immediately to Vilunya's request that she read the poem at the cremation. We would have a program then, a structure for the destruction of the corporeal Marty, a poem, a song, a ceremony that would have delighted Marty's anthropologist heart.

The small gothic chapel building was on the perimeter of Mount Auburn Cemetery, where, we were told, Longfellow is buried. The room, correctly called a crematorium, a word that sent a spasm of revulsion through me, was not quite ready for us. We were asked to wait outside until we were called. It was chilly on that early August morning. Our little group shifted from foot to foot and nervously studied the hastily copied words to La Martiniana. Finally, the room was ready, a workman told us in a kindly voice.

We shuffled hesitantly into the crematorium, each of us scanning the faces of the others, looking for signs of cracking, looking to see where help might be needed. A large cardboard box containing Marty in a plastic bag, rested on a gurney in front of the doors to the oven. Several of us took the lid off the box and I unzipped the bag. Marty's eyes had been closed. His skin felt like wax. I muttered, "Goodbye, Marty," and caressed his face for the last time.

And so, Margarita read the mournful, political poem in a strong, quick voice, and then, in enfeebled voices rendered off key by tears, we sang La Martiniana and slowly pushed him along the rollers into the oven and closed the doors behind him. A flutter went through me, a probe that sought out the parts of me beginning to hollow, the parts shared by Marty and me and now deserting me, gone with Marty. I was weak and incomplete. I wept helplessly, without sound, my shoulders slumped and my hands hanging lifelessly at my sides. Rodrigo, standing next to me, embraced me and I wept into his strong, young body.

Later, I sat alone with a glass of rum, trying to imagine what my life would be without Marty. Could memory replace the void? If it couldn't, how could I live with this emptiness? In the embrace of crushing fatigue and the too-relaxing effect of the alcohol, I thought of memory as matter, as palpable material that could be pumped into my voids as filler. I conjured Latin American images, symbols, modes of remembering. Marty is in the mountains, astride his white horse, Relampago, awaiting the call of his people, or, Marty is a luminescence, having cast off his human shell. I thought of the graffiti I had seen throughout Central America. Scrawled clandestinely across walls are the names of beloved figures, those who died defending their people: revolutionaries, priests, generals, visionaries. They appear like black wounds hastily inflicted upon whitewashed walls, the paint dripping from the bottom of the letters or neatly stenciled in the middle of the night. They simply say, Carlos Fonseca lives, Padre Romero is present, Sandino lives. They become part of history. They do not fade from memory. That is how it would be with me. It would not be as if something died in me, but rather, that I would now carry Marty within me, not as a painful burden, but as a weightless, inseparable, joyous part of me, till I died. Marty lives.

What bullshit, I told myself, angrily. Marty is dead. Dead is dead. He's gone forever and I remain without him. I don't need to idealize him, to invent a phony structure within which to worship him. I'll always feel him, I'll always remember him. He'll live for me within the ache of memory. But what will I be, what will this thing, this Saul, be, without the other part? Will the emptiness ever be filled? I heard the wild moan of the little boy, crying in a voice I didn't recognize, maybe the child's voice of the twins, begging to know, "Where's Marty, where's Sauly?"

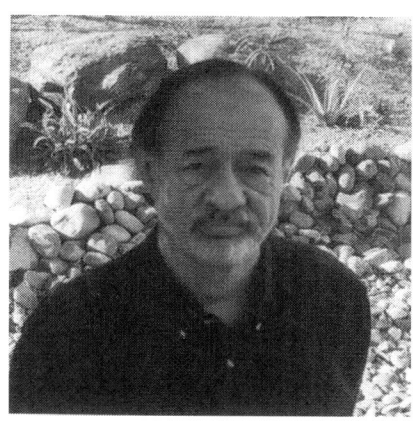

AUTHOR BIOGRAPHY

Saul Diskin, a retired businessman, lives in Arizona with his wife, Arline. They have three children and six grandchildren. A lifelong private writer, this is his first book. A second non-fiction book will follow shortly and a third, a novel, is nearing completion.

Printed in Great Britain
by Amazon

41795679R00158